The Complete Idiot's Refer...

What Is Your Sleep Per...

In this book, you'll not only find lots of tips on getting a good night's sleep in general, you'll also discover some interesting—and highly individual—facts about your unique sleep patterns and challenges. In Chapter 5, we offer a series of quizzes to help you identify your true sleep personality in more detail and in more categories. In the meantime, check off the statements you feel apply to you and see just what species of "sleep bird" you might be.

Are You a Lark?

____ The last time I managed to stay up to see Leno, he was Johnny Carson.

____ Morning is the very best time of my day.

____ Ben Franklin wrote "Early to bed, early to rise..." for people just like me.

Are You an Owl?

____ Nighttime is the right time—for just about anything!

____ The thought of a "breakfast club" sets my teeth on edge.

____ I have never met a midnight I didn't love.

Are You a Regular Robin?

____ I'm a pretty happy citizen of the 9-to-5 world—at least when it comes to its sleep and wake-up times.

____ To the occasional late night or early morning challenge, I can say: "No problem."

____ In my opinion, Larks who get up really early and Owls who stay up way past midnight just aren't "normal."

alpha books

Your Sleep/Wake Graph

To help determine just when and for how long you sleep, photocopy the following weeks' worth of the Sleep/Wake graph so that you can fill in a new one every day for at least a week or two. (See Chapter 5 for more information about how to fill out the graphs and what the patterns they reveal about your Sleep Personality and potential sleep problem.)

Your Sleep/Wake Graph

Monday
Work ....
Free ....
Sleep ....
12am 1 2 3 4 5 6 7 8 9 10 11 12pm 1 2 3 4 5 6 7 8 9 10 11 12am

Tuesday
Work ....
Free ....
Sleep ....
12am 1 2 3 4 5 6 7 8 9 10 11 12pm 1 2 3 4 5 6 7 8 9 10 11 12am

Wednesday
Work ....
Free ....
Sleep ....
12am 1 2 3 4 5 6 7 8 9 10 11 12pm 1 2 3 4 5 6 7 8 9 10 11 12am

Thursday
Work ....
Free ....
Sleep ....
12am 1 2 3 4 5 6 7 8 9 10 11 12pm 1 2 3 4 5 6 7 8 9 10 11 12am

Friday
Work ....
Free ....
Sleep ....
12am 1 2 3 4 5 6 7 8 9 10 11 12pm 1 2 3 4 5 6 7 8 9 10 11 12am

Saturday
Work ....
Free ....
Sleep ....
12am 1 2 3 4 5 6 7 8 9 10 11 12pm 1 2 3 4 5 6 7 8 9 10 11 12am

Sunday
Work ....
Free ....
Sleep ....
12am 1 2 3 4 5 6 7 8 9 10 11 12pm 1 2 3 4 5 6 7 8 9 10 11 12am

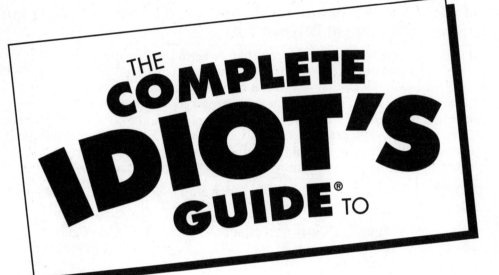

THE COMPLETE IDIOT'S GUIDE® TO

Getting a Good Night's Sleep

By Dr. Martin Moore-Ede and Suzanne LeVert

alpha books

A Division of Macmillan General Reference
A Simon & Schuster Macmillan Company
1633 Broadway, New York, NY 10019-6785

Macmillan Publishing books may be purchased for business or sales promotional use. For information please write: Special Markets Department, Macmillan Publishing USA, 1633 Broadway, New York, NY 10019.

International Standard Book Number: 0-02862394-0
Library of Congress Catalog Card Number: 98-86099

00 99 98   8 7 6 5 4 3 2 1

Interpretation of the printing code: the rightmost number of the first series of numbers is the year of the book's printing; the rightmost number of the second series of numbers is the number of the book's printing. For example, a printing code of 98-1 shows that the first printing occurred in 1998.

Printed in the United States of America

Note: This publication contains information based on the research and experience of its authors and is designed to provide useful advice with regard to the subject matter covered. The authors and publisher are not engaged in rendering medical or other professional services in this publication. Circumstances vary for practitioners of the activities covered herein, and this publication should not be used without prior consultation from a competent medical professional.

The authors and publisher expressly disclaim any responsibility for any liability, loss, injury, or risk, personal or otherwise, which is incurred as a consequence, directly or indirectly, of the use and application of any of the contents of this book.

Alpha Development Team

Publisher
Kathy Nebenhaus

Editorial Director
Gary M. Krebs

Managing Editor
Bob Shuman

Marketing Brand Manager
Felice Primeau

Senior Editor
Nancy Mikhail

Development Editors
Phil Kitchel
Jennifer Perillo
Amy Zavatto

Assistant Editor
Maureen Horn

Production Team

Book Producer
Lee Ann Chearney
Amaranth

Development Editor
Nancy Gratton

Production Editor
Christina Van Camp

Copy Editor
Lynn Northrup

Cover Designer
Mike Freeland

Photo Editor
Richard H. Fox

Illustrator
Jody P. Schaeffer

Designer
Kevin Spear

Indexer
Tim Wright

Layout/Proofreading
Angela Calvert
Mary Hunt

Contents at a Glance

Contents

Foreword

Sleep: It's an activity we all try to perform every day, just like eating or getting some exercise. So you might be surprised that the subject of sleep has been the official business of the United States Congress on more than one occasion. But you shouldn't be.

In fact, I first met the author of this book, Dr. Martin Moore-Ede, when he testified before the Subcommittee on Railroads of the House Committee on Transportation and Infrastructure. He discussed the relationship between fatigue and railroad accidents—indeed, between sleep deprivation and accidents of all kinds. When you read these startling statistics yourself—including the fact that at least 100,000 traffic accidents and 1,500 fatalities are due to sleep deprivation every year—you'll see why the Subcommittee is so interested in this issue.

I'd always attributed the occasional fatigue and listlessness I've experienced during the last few years to my 16-hour workdays and hectic schedule in Washington and New York. And, as much as I hate to admit it, my wife's complaints about my snoring fell upon deaf ears. Then, as part of a comprehensive physical, I found out I was one of millions of Americans with Obstructive Sleep Apnea, a potentially serious medical condition that was impacting my and (indirectly) my wife's health.

Just a few weeks after starting treatment (and you'll read about the remarkable treatment available for this type of sleep disorder in Chapter 14), I felt more energetic, more focused, and healthier than I had in years. And so did my wife.

And that's why I'm so heartily recommending this book: to help all of you who now barely make it through your days awake to feel better and to protect yourself against accidents and other health problems because you're not getting enough sleep. Dr. Moore-Ede and Suzanne LeVert have written a book that could, in its own way, save lives. Sleep deprivation—including drowsy driving—is a national safety concern. In *The Complete Idiot's Guide to Getting a Good Night's Sleep*, you'll find:

➤ The facts about how much sleep you—as a unique individual—really need

➤ The costs—economic, physical, and psychological—of sleep deprivation

➤ Solutions to the most common sleep problems and disturbances

➤ Special advice targeted to the millions of you who work the night shift or travel across time zones

➤ Fascinating and practical information about sleep through the life cycle—including how and why we dream.

Before you get too tired to turn the pages, read this book. Here's to getting a good night's sleep, tonight and every night.

Representative Sherwood L. Boehlert

Representative Sherwood Boehlert, a veteran Congressman first elected in 1982, is a moderate Republican. He focuses on the three "E"s—economic development, education, and the environment—and has earned a national reputation for his independence. As a senior member of both the Science and Transportation committees, an area of his focus is on research into improving transportation safety and public health. The two, Congressman Boehlert maintains, are intimately related.

Introduction

I like to rise at 4:30 a.m.; a colleague likes to rise at 10 a.m. I am a social zombie after 9 p.m., while he gets a surge of energy at midnight. He needs 9 hours of sleep a night, and I need 6¹/₂. I find an afternoon nap the best way to recover from sleep deprivation. He finds it tough to nap but can sleep in until noon.

Sleep is a highly personal, individual thing. There is no fixed formula for how much sleep you need or when you need to obtain it. But you'd better find out what works for you, or your health, mood, productivity, and personal safety will suffer. Indeed, sleep deprivation has become an increasingly serious health and safety concern in our modern 24-hour society—a society that never seems to sleep.

By focusing upon these essential facts—that sleep is a highly individual matter and that the typical modern lifestyle places a low priority on sleep—we've been able to create a very unique and special book, one that differs from the other excellent books that have been written about sleep. Other books may focus on the fascinating research discoveries from the world of sleep, or the average results of studies of large groups of people. Unfortunately, such books have limited value in helping the average man or woman improve their sleep.

The truth is, you not only need to understand the basics about sleep and the biological clock that maintains your sleep/wake pattern, you also have to know who you are. Nothing is worse for your health and your sanity than trying to conform your body's needs to someone else's view of what constitutes a good night's sleep. Each of us has a unique Sleep Personality that requires us to develop a personal strategy for getting the sleep we need. We can do that only by tailoring general advice to our own individual biological needs and preferences. In this book, we help you do just that.

How to Use This Book

If you or someone you love is having a hard time getting enough sleep to feel rested and alert throughout the day, read on. We'll help you plot your own special course on the journey to a better night's sleep. As you can see from the following figure, this book will take you through a mini- "diagnostic" procedure through which you'll discover a great deal about your lifestyle, your sleep patterns, and—with any luck—the potential cause of your sleep problem. You'll find out what your natural rhythms are and how they affect your sleep patterns; how long you really need to sleep; how easily (or not so easily) you can nap; and if a medical problem might be causing your sleep problem. You'll discover that you fall in the very wide range of "Extraordinarily Normal" or "Remarkably Special" sleepers, and for those of you who fall into each category, we explain your particular sleep patterns and potential problems, and then offer you a host of tried-and-true solutions in Part 2. Certain sleep problems may require special—even medical—attention to resolve: If you have a clinical sleep disorder or a medical condition, for instance, we send you right to a health professional evaluation. If you work the night shift, on the other hand, you need different advice, which we offer you in Chapter 17. Indeed, it's our job to help you find out where you fit into the world of sleep and to give you some direction when it comes to taking the next step toward identifying appropriate and effective solutions to your sleep problem.

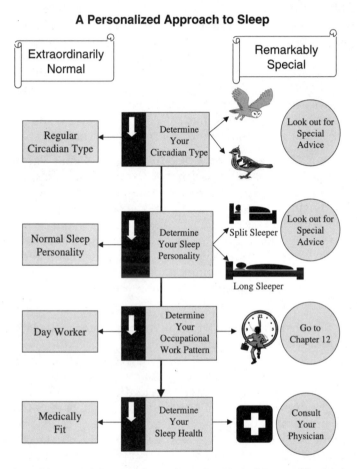

A Personalized Approach to Sleep

One size does not fit all when it comes to sleep. In this book, we take you through a set of quizzes so you can determine who you are and what help you may need. We will determine your circadian type, your sleep personality, and help you to understand your work-rest schedules and your sleep health. Based on your answers we will provide specially tailored advice.

Quite honestly, however, you may not find *all* the help you need here. If you're suffering from a serious sleep disorder or other medical problem, for instance, we suggest you get yourself to a doctor or specialist for advice and treatment.

That said, we give you the tools you need to determine your unique "Sleep Personality" and what that means to the way you approach your sleep problem. You'll find the most up-to-date information about the good sleep habits you'll want to foster and the bad habits you'll want to break, and we help you gain a better understanding of the most common sleep disorders (such as Obstructive Sleep Apnea and Restless Leg Syndrome) and disrupters (traveling across time zones and working the night shift).

We've divided the book into four parts, each exploring a different aspect of sleep. At the heart of every chapter, however, is a similar message: By better understanding both how you as an individual are meant to sleep and what in your life or your biology is keeping you awake, you'll be able to gain control over your sleep problem.

Part 1, "In the Arms of Morpheus," explores the basics of sleep. We start by explaining how little priority modern society places on sleep these days, and the medical and safety implications of sleep deprivation on an individual. We describe the internal body clock present in all humans (and most other living things) that maintains certain daily rhythms, including the sleep/wake cycle. Self-tests help you determine if you're getting enough sleep to stay awake and alert throughout the day and, if not, whether a medical problem might be causing your sleep problem. Then, in Chapter 5, we help you define your "Sleep Personality"—just how much sleep you really need and the best time (based on your lifestyle and your innate preferences) for you to obtain it.

After quizzing you about your sleep habits, Part 2, "Getting a Good Night's Sleep: Your Plan," outlines the basic sleep solutions that you can tailor to your own needs. We discuss how important having a proper diet, exercise routine, and stress reduction strategy is to getting a good night's sleep, and we describe the perfect sleep environment—one that's quiet, relaxing, and dark—that you should create in your own bedroom. Because we know how tempting the "quick fix" for your sleep problem may be, we also provide you with some facts and advice about using prescription and over-the-counter sleep remedies. We talk about how important exposure to bright light and pitch dark is to your sleep patterns, as well as how to nap (if you need to) during your natural daily dip in energy.

In Part 3, "Under Special Circumstances," you'll find all the basic information about the most common sleep disorders and disturbances. These include everything from snoring and sleep apnea to sleepwalking and teeth grinding. We also discuss problems that arise when your natural sleep/wake pattern, set by your internal body clock, becomes out-of-sync with your surroundings. This occurs in the sleep disorders called Delayed Phase Sleep Disorder (in which you can't get to sleep until quite early in the morning and can't get up until late in the day) and Advanced Phase Sleep Disorder (in which you can't stay up past 8 or 9 in the evening and wake up in the middle of the night). Jet lag, that all-too-common set of symptoms that occurs when you travel across time zones, and night shift work are two other types of sleep problems related to a mistimed body clock.

Part 4, "Sleep Through the Life Cycle," takes you through the stages of life, showing you how the need for sleep and the problems that can disrupt sleep develop as you age. From infancy to adolescence to middle age and late life, we describe common sleep patterns and what can go wrong to disrupt them. Our last chapter is devoted to dreaming, the seemingly magical way we spend about a quarter of our sleeping lives. Why do we dream? What do dreams really mean?

Extras

In addition to all of this helpful information organized into these four parts, we also provide sidebars throughout the text to explain unfamiliar terms, to further explore certain topics, or to give you helpful tips. Here's what to look for:

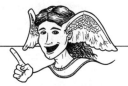

Morpheus Says

Factoids! Here, you'll read about interesting studies, statistics, and viewpoints relating to sleep, sleep research, and proper sleep hygiene.

Wake Up!

Warnings! The information provided in this sidebar warns you against certain behaviors that may disrupt your sleep or that otherwise work against getting a good night's sleep.

Just for You!

Occasionally throughout the book, we offer tidbits of information tailored to special needs of specific Sleep Personalities (Larks, Owls, Nappers and Non-Nappers, for instance). Once you determine your Sleep Personality, keep your eyes open for advice "Just for You."

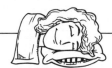

Sleep on it

Tips! Here we provide you with healthy suggestions and strategies that will improve your daily habits and help you get a better night's sleep.

Night Owl Wisdom

Definitions! Whenever we introduce an interesting or obscure word or term, we define it in one of these boxes.

Special Thanks from the Publisher to the Technical Reviewer

Our thanks to Dr. Pamela Valley Thacher, Ph.D. Dr. Thacher is currently a staff psychologist at Rhode Island Hospital in Providence. She received her doctoral degree in clinical psychology from the University of Connecticut and completed her internship and post-doctorate fellowship at Brown University's School of Medicine, specializing in the treatment of adult and adolescent sleep disorders. She recently gave birth to her first child, which has greatly expanded her knowledge of sleep deprivation.

Acknowledgments

We have lots of people to thank for helping us with this book, including, first and foremost, the dedicated staff members at Circadian Technologies who worked on this project: Acacia Aguirre, Ph.D., Ed Coburn, Anneke Heitmann, Ph.D., Steve Mardon, and Udo Trutschel, Ph.D. Without the expertise they thoughtfully and carefully offered—along with their healthy senses of humor and fun—this book could not have been written. The same can be said, as well, for Andrea DeCristofaro, whose patience and tenacity made the meetings among us possible. We'd also like to thank Lee Ann Chearney—book producer extraordinaire, thoughtful editor, and kind friend—for her help and support. To the people at Alpha Books, especially Kathy Nebenhaus, Gary Krebs, Bob Shuman, Nancy Gratton, and Chris Van Camp, we offer our thanks for their patience in us and their faith in the project.

Part 1

In the Arms of Morpheus

"Sleep? Who needs to sleep? You can sleep when you're dead."

Such a sentiment has led to a nation of sleep-deprived Americans barely able to get through the day, let alone feel well and fully alert.

What about you? Are you one of the millions of the sleep-deprived, putting yourself at increased risk of illness, accidents, or feeling just plain lousy? Do you even know how much sleep you really need? You'll find out when you read Part 1 and fill out the quizzes we provide in Chapters 4 and 5. Indeed, you'll have a brand new relationship with, and appreciation for, the world of sleep and your place in it.

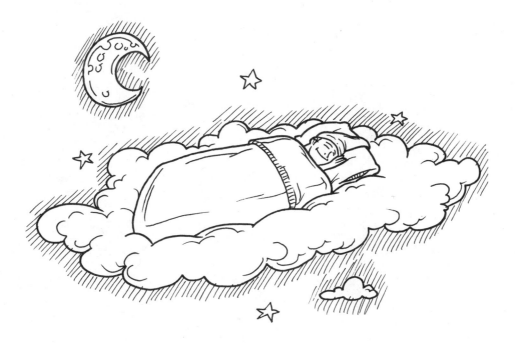

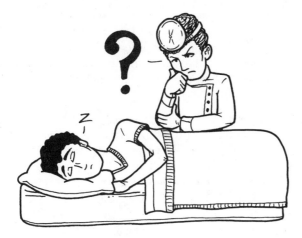

Chapter 1

What Is Sleep, Anyway?

In This Chapter

➤ The need for sleep

➤ Are you sleep deprived?

➤ The enemies of sleep

It seems like it should be the easiest thing in the world, doesn't it? Just lie back, close your eyes, and drift off into the blissful oblivion called sleep. Then, about 8 hours later, wake up feeling refreshed and renewed, ready to meet the challenge of staying awake and alert for the next 16 hours. That's the way it *should* work, right? Unfortunately, sleep isn't always that simple, nor is maintaining this standard sleep/wake schedule.

If you spend your nights tossing and turning instead of snoozing away, or if the demands of modern life interfere with a normal sleep schedule, you're far from alone. Lack of sleep is now a widespread modern problem: According to the National Sleep Foundation, nearly half of all Americans suffer from insomnia and other sleep-related disorders, and a recent Gallup survey reports that 56 percent of the adult population experience problems with daytime drowsiness. Indeed, lack of sleep has become a major health problem in the United States and around the world.

In this chapter, we'll help you better understand your biological need for sleep, and what can happen to your body when you go without it. We'll also outline the most common enemies of sleep, as well as help you determine if you're among the sleep deprived.

Sleep: A Modern Luxury

Fax machines transmit through the night. Television and computer screens defy darkness. Jets carry you across time zones in (practically speaking) the blink of an eye. Factories run all night. The world economy never sleeps and seems to expect the same of you.

The unfortunate fact of the matter, however, is that—like each of these man-made marvels—the human body has definite limits. Among those limits is the inability to run 24 hours a day, or even to easily revise our set patterns of sleep and wakefulness. And yet that's exactly what society expects from us—and what we believe we should expect from ourselves. "Sleep is a waste of time," the go-getters of the world seem to say. "You can sleep when you're dead." We hear that billionaire Donald Trump manages on just 3 to 4 hours, and President Clinton gets by on 4 or 5. If they can do it, so can we. In fact, we just better if we don't want to get left in the dust.

On the other hand, who can forget the sight of President George Bush, another notorious short sleeper and go-getter, vomiting on the podium in front of an official Japanese delegation? By staying up all day in Japan after traveling across several time zones, he'd forced his body beyond its capabilities. While most of us don't push ourselves to such extreme limits or experience such dramatic side effects from our struggles with sleep, every hour of rest we lose affects our health and well-being.

Without question, a primary factor when it comes to the current epidemic of sleep deprivation is the typical modern lifestyle of too much work, too much stimulation, and too little time. The technological advances of electricity and all those that followed from it now insist that we ignore a basic physiological need for regular periods of sleep in the darkness. If you work the night shift, either at your job or by caring for a family member at home, your problem is further compounded.

And then there's all the stuff you've got to fit into a mere Earth day: Working longer and longer hours to make ends meet; trying to spend time with your kids, your spouse, your ex, your in-laws; attempting to fit in a social life and some exercise. And goodness knows you just wouldn't feel on top of things if you didn't catch Letterman at midnight and the *Today Show* at dawn. When you get right down to it, you just don't have time to sleep.

Well, you better make time. Sleep is a basic biological need, every bit as essential to your health and well-being as food and water.

Night Owl Wisdom

Sleep deprivation is a term used to describe the state you're in when you do not obtain enough sleep to satisfy your body's needs.

The High Cost of Fatigue

Since you're reading this book, chances are you've spent a few sleepless nights yourself and know just how awful a night or two of poor sleep or no sleep can feel. From grouchiness to nausea to an inability to concentrate, the symptoms of *sleep deprivation* are uncomfortable and debilitating—and the side effects not only can interfere with your ability to enjoy a productive day, but are often deadly.

Just take a look at these shocking facts about sleep deprivation in the United States today:

➤ More than 30 percent of American drivers admit to having fallen asleep at the wheel at least once in their lifetime, and the National Sleep Foundation estimates that at least 100,000 accidents and 1,500 fatalities per year are due to falling asleep at the wheel.

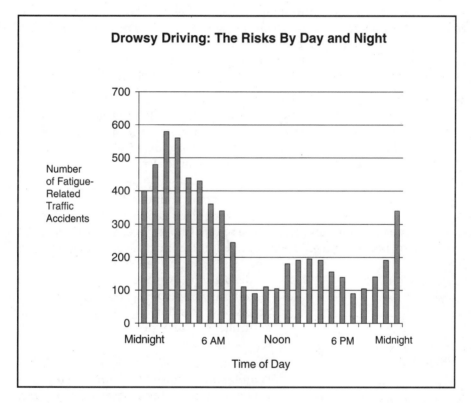

This graph is based on the results of several international studies involving more than 6,000 traffic accidents. As you can see, most drowsy driver accidents by far take place during the wee hours of the morning—between midnight and 6 a.m.—with another increase in mid-afternoon. And it's important to note that the proportion of traffic accidents related to fatigue at night is even higher, since fewer cars are on the road in the middle of the night.

After Mitler MM et al, Sleep 11: 100-109, 1988 with permission.

➤ The National Transportation Safety Board reported that "Fatigue is the No. 1 factor that detrimentally impacts the ability of pilots."

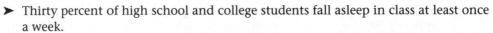

➤ Thirty percent of high school and college students fall asleep in class at least once a week.

➤ The direct costs of human fatigue to the American economy are about $70 billion per year—and worldwide, the figure may be as high as $300 billion.

Pretty big numbers, no? And all blamed on the lack of sleep, an essential physiological function most of us neglect. Indeed, sleep is probably the most underrated source of health and vitality available to the human race, one that we consistently ignore and discount. The consequences are not just economic, but very personal as well.

No doubt you already know how much a lack of sleep affects your ability to function. If you're running a power saw or performing a heart transplant when you're sleepy, the consequences can be fatal. But even if you're not involved in a potentially dangerous activity, sleep deprivation can be uncomfortable and upsetting. In addition to itchy eyes, which is the most universal symptom, several other physical problems arise:

➤ *Mood changes.* Irritability, depression, and anxiety are the three most common mood disturbances caused by lack of sleep. But we don't need to tell you that, do we? When you haven't satisfied your sleep needs, you're grouchy or miserable or twitchy (or maybe all three), aren't you? You also may feel overwhelmed and anxious facing even small challenges on too little sleep.

➤ *Decreased cognitive function.* Ever try to concentrate when you're sleep deprived, especially on something boring like balancing your checkbook or performing another routine task? If you're even a little sleep deprived, such tasks make you even sleepier, don't they? Ready to nod off? (In fact, you may well be nodding off: Many people who are sleep deprived suffer "microsleeps," brief episodes of sleep lasting only a few seconds.) Mistakes get made, big time, by the sleep deprived, which can get mighty dangerous if your job is tracking planes across busy corridors in the sky as an air-traffic controller or watching children play near the deep end of the pool.

➤ *Decreased motor skills.* Same goes here. Hand-eye coordination just isn't the same when you don't get enough sleep. And neither are your reflexes— the semi-automatic moves you make under certain circumstances, like braking or swerving when you see a puppy run out in front of your car.

➤ *Weight gain.* Yup. Not sleeping is definitely a risk factor when it comes to gaining weight. Think about it: What do you reach for when you're overtired? A candy bar, a soft drink, a doughnut— any quick high-carbohydrate, high-sugar food to give you a boost when you're dragging. Unfortunately, not only will this approach backfire and

Wake Up!

A sleep problem is a common symptom of depression, anxiety, and a wide variety of physical ailments including diabetes, asthma, and arthritis. That's why it's important to see your doctor to rule out other causes for your sleep difficulties or chronic fatigue. You may need treatment for the underlying illness as well as for your difficulties with sleep.

leave you feeling more tired than ever, but if your sleep problem is chronic, you'll start gaining weight as those snacks pile up.

➤ *Impaired immune system.* It isn't your imagination: You really do run a greater risk of getting a cold or other infection when you lack sleep. We now know that lack of sleep undermines your immune system's ability to fight off foreign intruders like viruses and bacteria.

As you can see, you need to sleep well on a regular basis in order to maintain your health and function with relative efficiency and safety in your daily life. But why, exactly, is that true? What *is* sleep, anyway?

Sleep: The Final Frontier

To be able to sleep, and sleep well, isn't as easy as it sounds. In fact, sleep is a downright complex behavior, involving a wide range of physiological activities. You fall asleep and then wake up as your body temperature falls and rises in a distinct pattern. Hormones secreted by various endocrine glands help set up the internal environment for periods of sleep and wakefulness, working with your brain in a delicate and intricate dance throughout the day and night.

The key to this process is the internal body clock, which each of us inherits from our parents along with our other unique attributes. As we'll discuss further in chapters 2 and 5, your body has a rhythm all its own, and left to its own devices would "choose" to sleep a specific amount of time at certain times of the day. Understanding your own personal rhythm (which may differ from other people's) and learning to adapt it to a different schedule—occasionally or on an on-going basis—without becoming sleep deprived is essential to good health and a productive life.

The amount of stress in your life and your ability to cope with it, your diet, and your exercise habits also have a definite impact on how much and how well you sleep. Needless to say, it's often difficult to fall asleep when you're tense with worry and anxiety, or when too much caffeine stimulates the brain just when you want it to slow down. Although getting some exercise doesn't automatically mean a good night's sleep, people who exercise on a regular basis tend to suffer from less depression and anxiety, conditions that often disrupt sleep. Exercisers also tend not to be overweight, a risk factor for snoring and a breathing disorder called Obstructive Sleep Apnea, two other enemies of sleep.

In Part 3, "Sleep Solutions," you'll learn the fundamentals of proper sleep hygiene: what you need to change in your life and environment to prepare

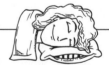

Sleep on it

If you have trouble sleeping and can't figure out why, try looking no further than the other side of your bed. Is your partner's tossing and turning, snoring and fidgeting, or chronic blanket snatching keeping you awake? If so, it may be time for one of you to sleep in the guest room until the problem is resolved.

your body and mind for sleep every night. In the meantime, it's important to understand just how damaging poor sleep can be.

What Sleep Is

We should know what sleep is, right? After all, over a lifetime of sleeping an average for 8 hours a night, a person who lives to be 75 years old will have slept approximately 219,000 hours. (Keep in mind, however, that this is just an average: Many people sleep far more or less than the "standard" 8 hours, and sleep patterns change dramatically from infancy to old age.) Without sleep, then, you could put in another 5,475 weeks of work (heaven forbid!) or watch the complete series of original *Star Trek* re-runs more than 2,730 times (any better?). Nevertheless, not even sleep researchers like myself fully understand the process and purpose of sleep.

Webster's New World Dictionary defines sleep this way: "A natural, regularly recurring condition of rest for the body and mind, during which the eyes are usually closed and there is little or no conscious thought or voluntary movement...." All in all, a pretty straightforward description. To break this definition down, sleep involves four observable criteria:

➤ *Stillness.* When we're asleep, we usually don't walk, talk, or perform other activities. The word *usually* is very important, as you'll see later. There are, in fact, people who stand at the refrigerator and scarf down a whole German chocolate cake and others who divulge state secrets to anyone within earshot—all while completely and utterly asleep.

➤ *Supine posture.* Generally speaking, humans sleep lying down or, when absolutely necessary, sitting down. With a few exceptions (see above), we can say that someone performing a headstand or washing the dishes is not asleep.

➤ *Unresponsiveness to low-level stimuli.* When you're asleep, your sensory "radar" is less finely tuned than when you're awake. You're not aware of Fido's foul breath (unless he wakes you up by panting directly into your nostrils) or of the gentle breeze wafting through the trees outside your window.

➤ *Reversibility.* The sound of an alarm clock or a little shake is usually all it takes to wake someone from even the deepest of sleeps. That quality differentiates sleep from coma or, say, death, both of which can look a lot like sleep to the amateur eye.

Of course, we sleep researchers also have some stricter physiological criteria by which we define sleep. We measure brain waves, eye movements, and muscle activity. Since the 1950s, researchers have studied distinct changes in brain waves, eye movements, and muscle tension, which vary between wakefulness and sleep, and also differ among the various stages of sleep.

As we'll discuss in further depth in Chapter 3, sleep is hardly a static, uniform activity, but rather has many layers and stages. The most important division is between REM and non-REM (NREM) sleeps. REM stands for *rapid eye movement*, because your eyes periodically move rapidly during that stage. It is also the stage during which you dream. Brain waves during REM sleep closely resemble those of wakefulness, but your muscles are almost paralyzed, thanks to the actions of a set of nerve cells deep within the brain.

Morpheus Says

Research suggests that that our muscles are in a state of near paralysis during the dreaming period of REM sleep to protect us against acting out our dreams. People with a condition called REM Behavior Disorder actually perform the actions they're dreaming about. One subject, dreaming (as so many men do) that he was playing professional football, tried to tackle the wall in front of him.

During NREM sleep, on the other hand, the body moves more naturally, such as when you reposition yourself in bed. It's also when most behaviors like sleepwalking and sleeptalking take place. Brain waves are much slower than they are during REM sleep, and eye movement pretty much ceases. Scientific research suggests that much of the rest and repair for which sleep is best known takes place during the NREM stage.

In order to get a good night's sleep, you must experience both REM and NREM sleep. What's really interesting is that we sleep in cycles of REM and NREM, each cycle lasting about 90 minutes, which means you go through four or five cycles per night and, potentially, have four or five different dreams to remember!

Birds Do It, Bees Do It...

And yes, even fleas and the dogs they live on do it. Sleep is a basic biological need of all mammals, and most other living things, including birds and reptiles. (Believe it or not, even plants appear to sleep, or rather have rhythms of activity and dormancy that roughly correlate to the sleep/wake behavior of animals.)

The study of sleep patterns in animals—worth a whole book all by itself—demonstrates the remarkable accommodations animals make in order to sleep. Take, for instance, whales and dolphins. These creatures actually sleep with just one half of their brain at a time, while the other half stays awake. Many species of birds also manage to sleep and fly at the same time using this same half-a-brain method.

Some animals sleep primarily at night (like us humans), whereas others retire during the day (rats and other rodents, which is a definite plus). Horses can sleep standing up, their leg muscles remaining taut and strong enough to hold up their weight. However, horses do most of their sleeping in a much more comfortable, supine position.

Cats, of course, are special for lots of reasons: Their elegance, their snuggability, and their quirky personalities. What's truly amazing, however, is their capacity for sleep. The average pussycat sleeps at least 12 to 14 hours per day, in no apparent rhythm. (And they say it's a dog's life!)

You can see from this brief rundown of animal behavior that sleep is an integral part of life on planet Earth, no matter what the species. However, the question remains: exactly why do we sleep a third of our lives away?

The Benefits of Sleep

Why is sleep so important? What function does it serve to the human body and mind? Unfortunately, no one really knows the precise answers to these questions. There are, however, many different theories.

➤ *Rest.* It seems pretty obvious that one reason we sleep—perhaps the main reason—is that sleep helps to "recharge" our physical and psychological batteries. At the same time, however, we know that certain parts of brain work harder during sleep than during wakefulness. So providing us with rest is not the whole sleep story. Indeed, feeling fatigued after a hard day's work is only one of the reasons we fall asleep; automatic changes in body temperature and hormone levels have a lot to do with it, too.

➤ *Growth and repair.* Sleep appears to help body cells grow and regenerate. During deep sleep in the early part of the night, the endocrine system secretes human growth hormone (HGH), a body chemical that stimulates the growth of muscle and organ tissues. During adulthood, the hormone acts to trigger the repair of these tissues.

➤ *Energy conservation.* When you're awake, your body burns a great deal of oxygen and food to provide energy for daily physical and mental activities. Called "catabolism," this process burns up your energy reserves. During sleep, your body is more anabolic, meaning it conserves energy. For instance, when you're asleep, both your body temperature and your metabolism (the rate at which you burn energy) falls. In essence, sleep gives the body a break from its daily physiological activities.

➤ *Memory consolidation and discharge of emotions.* Some researchers believe that sleep helps reinforce memories, whereas dreaming—a natural part of the sleep process—helps sort and purge deep-seated emotional issues. We'll talk more about dreams and their possible role in our mental and physical health in Chapter 23.

➤ *Safety.* In many mammals, sleep offers respite from food chain activity. In other words, a mouse asleep in its burrow is unlikely to attract the attention of a prowling, hungry cat. Even humans are safer, for the most part, when they're asleep in their own beds than when they're awake and crossing the street against the light or even going up and down the stairs at home.

What Can Go Wrong

Okay, now you know why you might need sleep and how universal the need is among earthly creatures. But if you're reading this book, you probably don't know how to get enough of it. As we told you at the beginning of this chapter, you're not alone in your struggle for a good night's sleep.

For most Americans, the enemies of sleep are found in our lifestyle. We're too busy, stressed, underexercised, and overweight to sleep well. In other cases, medical sleep disorders interfere with proper sleep. In Chapter 4, you'll learn about those disorders and then, in Part 3, some of the solutions that can help alleviate them. In the meantime, here's a quick rundown of the most common enemies:

➤ *Insomnia.* Insomnia is a general term for a variety of problems having to do with getting and staying asleep. Literally, the word *insomnia* means "no sleep" during a 24-hour period, but most people who suffer with insomnia get at least some sleep. Insomnia can be transient (lasting only a night or two on an occasional basis), short-term (lasting from three nights to three weeks), or chronic (long-lasting and intransigent). In some cases, insomnia can be traced to a medical problem; in others, a lifestyle issue; and in still others, no cause can be found. Chapter 6 helps guide you through the world of sleeplessness known as insomnia.

➤ *Disruption of sleep patterns.* Sometimes for no known reason, sometimes because of shift work or travel across time zones, your sleep patterns become disrupted. You fall asleep and wake up too early or too late to keep company with the world around you. Such problems usually require the help of a sleep specialist to solve. In Chapters 16, 17, and 18, we discuss such disturbances in more depth.

➤ *Snoring and sleep apnea* (yours or your partner's). Author Anthony Burgess once wrote, "Laugh and the world laughs with you; snore and you snore alone." Simple snoring not only interferes with your partner's sleep, but also often disrupts your ability to sleep deeply yourself. Its close relative Obstructive Sleep Apnea is even more serious. Sleep apnea causes breathing to stop from 10 seconds up to a minute at a time, after which you wake up for a few seconds or minutes, often gasping for breath, and then fall back asleep—sometimes without ever realizing you've been disturbed. We discuss snoring and sleep apnea, and some solutions to them, in Chapter 14.

➤ *Parasomnias* (yours or your partner's). Walking and talking after midnight can be sexy, sweet pastimes—as long as you're not actually sound asleep while you're doing them. Teeth-grinding and night terrors (startling, upsetting partial or total awakenings from deep sleep) are other parasomnias. Other disturbing disorders include Restless Leg Syndrome, which is characterized by discomfort in the legs relieved by movement, and Periodic Limb Movements in Sleep, characterized by sporadic leg movements or jerks. Clearly, both can wreak havoc on sleep for anyone who happens to be in the bed. We explain these problems in more depth in Chapter 15.

➤ *Medical illness.* Infections, allergies, pain, indigestion, and many other medical conditions have sleep problems as side effects. In addition, the drugs you take to treat these and other illnesses may also cause insomnia.

➤ *Emotional disturbances.* A recent divorce, the death of a loved one, work pressures, a bout of the blues: Any of these emotional difficulties—commonly lumped together under the heading of "stress"—can interfere with your ability to get to sleep and stay asleep. The solutions we discuss in Part 2 can help someone with a temporary emotional upset get better sleep.

How Much Sleep *Do* You Need?

It's true that the *average* adult seems to exist on about 7¹/₂ hours of sleep. That's not to say, however, that 7¹/₂ hours is the standard amount of sleep we need or even desire. Some sleep studies show that, given their druthers, many people would choose to sleep about 8 to 9 hours on a regular basis. The fact that most of us consistently get less than that shows just how widespread sleep deprivation has come to be.

That said, sleep requirements and preferences are highly individual things. They vary from person to person, under different circumstances, and at different times of life. Generally speaking, though, there are at least four categories of sleep behavior:

➤ *Long sleepers vs. short sleepers.* Some people need those 9 or 10 hours of sleep in order to feel well, while others thrive on just 5 or 6.

➤ *Rigid sleepers vs. flexible sleepers.* Some people wake up at the same time every morning no matter what time they go to bed, even if they've slept only a few hours. Others can easily adjust their sleep patterns to accommodate changes in their normal social or work schedules.

➤ *Larks vs. owls.* No doubt you've heard of this category already: The morning people and the night people…those who do their best work at the crack of dawn and those who don't really come alive until evening.

➤ *Nappers vs. non-nappers.* Some people are able to make up for lost sleep time by taking a nap, whereas others simply have to exist through the day until their next nocturnal sleep period. Dedicated nappers find that a daily nap becomes an essential part of their sleep/wake pattern, and that they don't function as well on days when they miss that afternoon snooze.

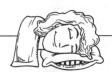

Sleep on it

Don't assume you have a sleep problem if you sleep more or less than the average 7¹/₂ hours a night. If you wake up feeling refreshed and alert, and function well during the day, on a regular basis, chances are you're getting just the right amount of sleep for you.

In Chapter 5, you'll discover what your "Sleep Personality" is, and how it affects your ability to get enough regular sleep. You'll also learn how to keep a "Sleep Log" so that you'll know exactly how much sleep you get and how you feel at various times during the day. We'll also help you to understand how your work, family, and social life affect your sleep patterns and how to make the most out of the schedule you have today.

Is it possible to exist on 4, 5, or 6 hours of sleep a night? Absolutely. As long as you wake up feeling rested, and remain alert throughout the day, you'll be just fine. Are you ill if you need to sleep 9 or 10 hours a day? Not at all. Consider this: We estimate that the average person 100 years ago, before the electric light bulb ruled the night, slept about 8 to 9 hours. Today, the average person sleeps just $7^1/_2$ hours a night—and millions complain of feeling chronically tired and out of sorts.

Do you believe that you sleep enough and feel rested when you wake up? Or is it possible that you are among the millions of sleep-deprived walking the streets of America today? The following quiz will help you determine your sleep status.

Are You Getting Enough?

1. I wish I had more energy.
   Yes ___ No ___

2. I frequently have a headache in the morning.
   Yes ___ No ___

3. I often have to struggle during the day to remain alert.
   Yes ___ No ___

4. I often have trouble concentrating.
   Yes ___ No ___

5. I seem to tire easily when performing physical tasks.
   Yes ___ No ___

6. I seem to be particularly susceptible to colds and other infections.
   Yes ___ No ___

7. I often feel like I'm going to fall asleep while driving.
   Yes ___ No ___

8. I often feel like I'm in a daze.
   Yes ___ No ___

9. My friends and family say that I tend to be often grumpy and irritable.
   Yes ___ No ___

10. I worry about things and have trouble relaxing.
    Yes ___ No ___

If you've answered more than three or four of these questions with a yes, you may be able to trace your difficulty to a sleep problem. At the same time—and we'll say this more than once in this book—these same behaviors and symptoms may indicate a physical or psychological problem that requires treatment or advice from a medical doctor. If you're having chronic sleep problems, you should make an appointment with your doctor for a check-up to rule out other causes.

The Strength of Sleep

The good news is that for almost every common sleep problem, there is a solution. Some solutions involve making lifestyle changes, like cutting back on caffeine or changing your diet. Severe cases of sleep apnea and disturbances of the body clock may require more intensive treatment.

That's not to say that every case of insomnia is easily fixable—some can be maddeningly stubborn and the underlying cause of the problem difficult to identify. But with patience, effort, and a little trial and error, sleep may cease to be so tantalizingly out of reach.

Read on, and we'll help you figure out what's keeping you up at night and find a way to get you a good night's sleep and thus feel more vital, alert, and alive.

The Least You Need to Know

➤ Chronic sleep deprivation is a dangerous and debilitating condition.

➤ It's possible to be sleep deprived and not realize it.

➤ There is a solution to almost every sleep problem, probably even yours.

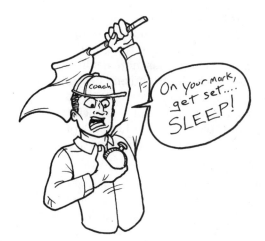

Chapter 2

Timing Is Everything

In This Chapter

➤ Identifying the internal clock

➤ Mapping the daily cycles of life

➤ Understanding your personal rhythms

Choices: You've got a lot of them to make every day, don't you? What time to get up, when to exercise, what to eat and when, how hard to work. For the most part, you have the power to choose how you live—at least within the context of the 20th century social imperatives of work and family life. Such decisions are completely yours to make, or so it seems.

You might be surprised, however, how much a powerful internal mechanism known as the biological clock influences your desires and abilities. This clock sets up a pattern for your daily life that you follow in more ways than you realize. In this chapter, we'll explore the way the biological clock works, how it was discovered, and what it means to your sleep patterns and other daily rhythms.

Tick, Tock, Your Internal Clock

There are only 24 hours in the day, right? Well, actually, that depends on what kind of day you're talking about. The Earth does indeed make a complete rotation on its axis about every 24 hours and circles around the sun every 365¼ days. Our civilization has constructed a clock and a calendar based on this regular cycle of light/dark and change of season.

But we now know that the human body has its own way of keeping time that's al-most—but not quite—in harmony with this rhythm of nature and the very rigid man-made clock we've developed to keep track of it. Your internal (or *endogenous*) clock is far more flexible than the one that ticks on your nightstand and desktop and is far more individual. In fact, you have a slightly different internal rhythm than does anyone else—which may explain why your boss seems to be at her peak of efficiency at 8 a.m., while you're still wiping sleep dust from your eyes!

Night Owl Wisdom

Endogenous is a word used to describe a rhythm or condition that arises within the body and is not caused or triggered by external or environmental factors.

Although the differences between your internal clock and the man-made one, and between your natural rhythms and those of the people around you, might be small, those differences can strongly affect how you feel mentally, emotionally, and physically.

Your Sleep/Wake Rhythm

So exactly what does your endogenous clock keep track of and help to coordinate? Pretty much every biological activity you can think of, from your body temperature to the hormones that course through your bloodstream to how often your stomach contracts. In turn, these biological events profoundly influence the way you behave and how you feel as you go about your daily routine.

You probably know, for instance, that the average "normal" body temperature for humans is about 98.6°F. What you might not realize is that your temperature fluctu-ates in a set pattern on a daily basis. Your temperature is at its low point (about 96°F) between 4 a.m. and 6 a.m., then climbs sharply during the morning hours and more gently during the afternoon. It reaches its peak of about 99°F between 7 p.m. and 8 p.m., and then begins to fall to its low point once again.

Night Owl Wisdom

The **suprachiasmatic nuclei,** or **SCN,** is a tiny cluster of brain cells that acts as the body's primary biological clock. It helps orchestrate the sleep/wake cycle and a host of other physiological functions.

Experiments show that the body temperature cycle and the sleep/wake cycle are normally intimately linked: We feel more alert the higher our body temperature is (within normal limits!), and our energy and ability to concentrate tend to sag the lower the temperature falls.

Another key biological rhythm when it comes to the sleep/wake cycle is the secretion of a hormone called melatonin. The pineal gland, an endocrine organ located in the brain, releases melatonin synchronized by a signal from the *suprachiasmatic nuclei (SCN)*. Melatonin and body temperature rise and fall in a mirror image, together setting the stage for sleep. As the body tempera-ture falls, the level of melatonin rises, and we begin to feel sleepy. As the temperature rises, melatonin levels fall, and we wake up. Other hormones rise and fall in a regular pattern as well: Levels of the stress hormones that ready our bodies for action, such as cortisol, start to rise as melatonin falls, stimulating us to wake up ready to face the day.

Of course, sleep can, and does, occur at all phases of the day. But how well and how long you sleep depends a great deal on *when* you go to sleep. In fact, there are at least two "preferred" times for sleep within the 24-hour period: 1) the major one that occurs at night as the body temperature is falling (and melatonin levels rising) and 2) one that occurs just after lunch, from around 1 to 3 in the afternoon. The afternoon sleep period rarely lasts more than an hour and a half in adults. This desire for an afternoon siesta is part of many cultures. And, just as there are preferred times for sleep, there is also a so-called "forbidden zone": Many people find it almost impossible to fall asleep between the hours of 7 and 9 p.m., for example, although as you'll see in Chapter 5, aspects of your Sleep Personality (what time you naturally prefer to go to bed and get up, to nap or not, and how long you sleep) play a role in the exact timing of your "preferred" and "forbidden zones" for sleep.

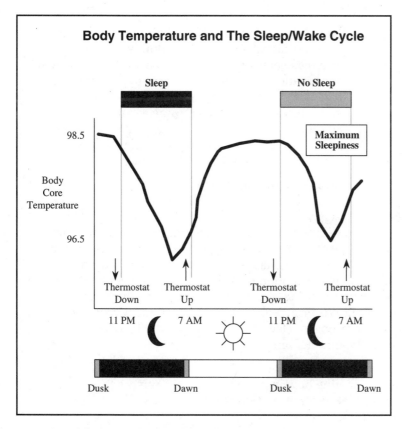

As you can see from this graph, your body temperature—triggered by your internal body clock—starts falling as the night begins (setting the stage for sleep) and then begins to rise in the hours before dawn (helping get you ready for the day ahead). What's interesting is that this circadian rhythm of temperature rise and fall occurs whether or not you go to sleep.

Accordingly, if no one told you how to plan your day, then you'd probably find that you're better able to concentrate on complex tasks in the morning, that you crave a nap in mid-afternoon, and that you feel pretty strong while exercising at about 5 p.m. Within an hour or two before midnight you'd be ready for a major sleep period. That's because your biological clock has set these rhythms in motion. You can work around them if you have to (as most of us do on a fairly routine basis), or your own rhythms may be different enough to put you a few hours ahead or behind (we'll talk about "morning people" and "night people" later in the chapter and more specifically in Chapter 5). But all things being equal, most people would take a nap in mid-afternoon and go to bed before midnight.

Rhythms, Rhythms Everywhere

Because many of the body's activities occur in a 24-hour cycle, but may drift out of synch with local day and night on occasion, one of the early researchers in this area, Dr. Franz Halberg of the University of Minnesota, named them *circadian* (Latin for "about a day") rhythms.

Night Owl Wisdom

The term **circadian** is taken from the Latin *circa*, which means "about," and *dies*, which means "day." Circadian rhythms are those biological rhythms that recur about every 24 hours.

Daily, or circadian rhythms, aren't the only internal patterns that exist in the body, however. Rhythms that are longer than a day (called infradian rhythms) include menstruation, and those that recur in periods shorter than a day (called "ultradian rhythms") include certain hormone secretions and—most relevant to this book—our nightly sleep patterns that last about 90 minutes each. As we'll discuss later, this 90-minute cycle also influences our state of alertness throughout the day.

Circannual rhythms, such as hibernation and migration, exist throughout the animal world. Though we humans usually consider ourselves too "highly evolved" for such events, we also have some unmistakable circannual rhythms: Secretion of the male hormone testosterone surges in the fall, sperm concentration and activity is highest in the winter, and rates of conception peak in winter as well. So it follows that more babies are born in August and September than in any other month. A seasonal pattern for death exists as well: We die at a much higher rate in the winter—and it isn't just because of the cold. Even people in Hawaii and Florida have higher death rates in the winter months than in the summer ones.

By now you're probably wondering exactly what this internal clock looks like and where it is in the body. Considering how important it is to the way we live our lives, it might surprise you to know that its discovery was fairly recent, and there's still a lot we don't know about how it works.

The Primary Pacemaker

In 1972, two independent groups of scientists led by Irving Zucker and Robert Moore made an important discovery: They identified a small cluster of about 10,000 neurons (nerve cells) within the brains of rats called the suprachiasmatic nuclei (SCN). This tiny clump of cells, which my colleagues and I located in the human brain in 1980, serves as the body's primary biological clock, a powerful pacemaker that coordinates the body's rhythms.

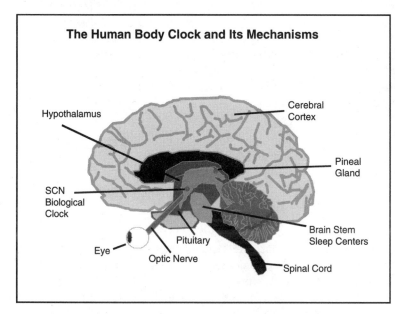

The Human Body Clock and Its Mechanisms

Hypothalamus

Cerebral Cortex

Pineal Gland

SCN Biological Clock

Brain Stem Sleep Centers

Eye

Pituitary

Optic Nerve

Spinal Cord

What keeps your body running in a regular, approximately 24-hour rhythm is the suprachiasmatic nuclei (the SCN), a cluster of cells located in the center of the brain. The SCN receives information about night and day from the optic nerve, which transmits dark and light information from the eyes. When it's dark, the SCN then stimulates the pineal gland to release melatonin, a hormone that sends its own messages to the body about sleep, and triggers the brain stem sleep centers.

The discovery of the SCN was just one step in a very long journey that continues today. It started as early as the 4th century B.C., when Alexander the Great's scribe Androsthenes noticed that certain plants had leaves that opened up during the day and then closed at night in a robust and predictable pattern. This pattern appeared to follow the rise and fall of the sun. Over 2,000 years later, Androsthenes' observation led to the creation of a whole new science called chronobiology, the study of biological rhythms.

For centuries, humans assumed that the rising and setting of the sun acted as the sole trigger for such rhythmic activity. Then, in 1729, French astronomer Jean Jacques d'Ortous de Mairan performed a simple but elegant experiment that forever confounded that notion: He left a Mimosa plant in a dark closet and watched as it continued to open its leaves in the morning and close them up again at night—despite having no exposure to the cyclic rising and setting of the sun. This activity led de Mairan to conclude that leaf behavior originated within the plant itself and that sunlight played little or no role in maintaining the pattern.

For more than 100 years, the study of biological rhythms remained largely in the hands of botanists; other species, including humans and other mammals, didn't come under scrutiny until 1866. At that time, William Ogle made careful observations about the pattern of body temperature in humans. In his own words, "There is a rise in the early morning while we are still asleep, and a fall in the evening while we are still awake, which cannot be explained by…variations in light." In 1910, Swiss physician August Forel observed a circadian rhythm in the behavior of worker bees: After first noticing the bees sampling some marmalade left out on a picnic table after breakfast, he watched as the bees arrived each morning just before breakfast time, as if they knew when to expect food. Then, in 1919, Curt Richter, a young researcher at Johns Hopkins University School of Medicine, began a lifelong quest to understand what made rats, humans, and other mammals tick. Through hundreds of studies, he charted the natural patterns of sleeping, eating, drinking, and exercising in several different species. This work continues in laboratories all over the world today.

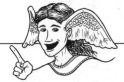

Morpheus Says

An interesting contribution to the science of chronobiology came from Carolus Linneaus, the eighteenth century botanist and taxonomist. After determining the time at which certain flowers opened and closed their petals, he devised a charming "clock garden." He placed clusters of particular flowers in positions representing the hours of the day, and thus by seeing which flower petals had opened, he could tell the approximate time of day.

What Richter and his colleagues past and present have determined is that all animals—humans included—have internal rhythms of behavior and physiology that persist under all sorts of circumstances—in constant light or darkness, with or without access to food, interrupted by noise or in total silence. What maintains these rhythms are internal biological clocks, including the SCN, that pulsate in regular rhythms. These clocks send out signals that control a host of behaviors, such as when to wake up, go to sleep, eat, and mate.

Not until after World War II, however, was it known if the human body—like the Mimosa plant—would maintain these regular rhythms without the aid of sunlight or other environmental stimuli. It took putting volunteers into "time-free" environments almost like the dark closet that served as the Mimosa plant's temporary home to make this discovery.

Tracking Internal Time

Nathaniel Kleitman, a pioneer in sleep research, conducted one of the first human experiments showing the effects of isolation on human rhythms. He and a colleague isolated themselves in a continuously lit chamber in Mammoth Cave, Kentucky. Their aim was to remove themselves from all outside influences, including cycles of light and dark. Such studies are called "temporal isolation experiments" because they deprive the participants of outside stimuli that could otherwise influence their behavior. The participants' rhythms can thus run free of external influences, which is why the circadian rhythms in these experiments are called "free-running." German scientists Jurgen Aschoff and Rutger Wever created such a time-free environment in 1962 when they isolated individuals in a sealed cellar below a Munich hospital from 8 to 19 days. Over the next 20 years, researchers studied hundreds of people as they lived for a month or more in a specially built underground bunker—experiments that laid the foundation of human circadian physiology. Then, in the late 1970s, on the top floor of a New York Hospital, Elliot Weitzman, Charles Czeisler, and I built the first lab to study human sleep behavior in a time-free environment.

What we and the other researchers discovered is that the human body does not run exactly on a 24-hour day, but usually on a slightly longer schedule. Internal rhythms stay the same—body temperature rises and falls in a set pattern, for instance—but the pattern doesn't quite fit into the 24-hour day.

When it comes to the sleep/wake cycle, human participants in free-running experiments on average establish a day of about 24.8 hours, almost an hour longer than the regular day—although it's important to note that there is a wide-range of day lengths, typically from 24.2 hours to 25.5, depending on the individual and the conditions imposed by the study. Every day, then, bedtime shifts later by an extra hour, so that by two weeks into the experiment, most participants are about a half a day out of synchrony with the outside world. They sleep when the rest of society is up and about, and vice versa.

Sometimes in these isolation experiments, the sleep/wake cycle stretches out much longer to 30 to 40 hours, so that days appear to fly by at almost twice the normal speed. The subjects are amazed to find how much they have underestimated the passage of time when they finally emerge into the world.

Since the body clock naturally beats with a different rhythm from the man-made one—how are we able to exist in such coordination with the 24-hour day? After all, most of us live on the 16 hours up, 8 hours in bed routine, getting up around 7 a.m. and going to sleep by midnight, give or take a few hours either way.

The answer is light. Indeed, although our 4th century B.C. reporter Androsthenes didn't see the whole picture when he thought the sun caused the plants' leaves to open and close, the sun does play an important role in synchronizing human biological rhythms.

When isolated from external Zeitgebers (primarily the rising and setting of the sun), your body clock—and therefore your bedtime and wake-up time—naturally drifts later by an hour every day.

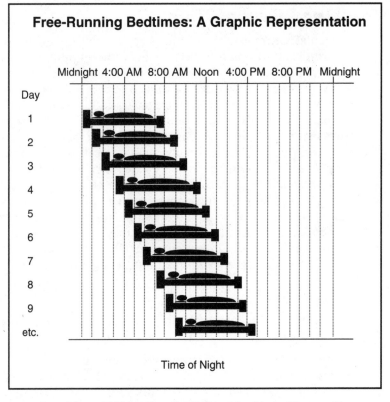

Free-Running Bedtimes: A Graphic Representation

Time of Night

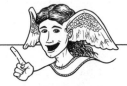

Morpheus Says

Does time really fly when you're having fun?

All studies of long-term time estimation have reported an average "subjective hour" of slightly longer than an hour—from just a few seconds to over 30 minutes longer. And time *doesn't* fly when you're having fun: In a study in which some people were encouraged to keep up their daily activities (reading, exercise, and writing, for example) and the others were prohibited from engaging in any activity, both groups estimated that the hour on average consisted of about 1.12 hours. Studies have also found that periods of sleep are underestimated to a greater extent than are intervals of wakefulness, regardless of the degree of activity during the waking bout. Sleep slows our perception of the passage of time.

Know Your Zeitgebers

The human biological clock—the SCN—is located right near the optic chiasm. The optic chiasm is the junction box where the pathways from the two eyes merge and cross over on their way to the brain, carrying visual information about the outside world, including information about light and dark. The SCN gathers information from a special bundle of nerves within the optic pathways and uses it to keep the body more or less synchronized—or *entrained*—to the environmental 24-hour cycle of light and dark. You can think of information about light and dark as a kind of force that nudges the biological clock and tries to keep it in step with the world around us.

Indeed, sunlight, or any light if it is bright enough, acts as the main timegiver, or *Zeitgeber*, for most species, although the location of light-sensitive cells aren't always where you might expect them. Horseshoe crabs, for instance, have light sensors on their tails, swallows have them just inside their skull, and fruit flies have time-keeping devices active in their legs, wings, and hair bristles, suggesting that their entire bodies are rigged to keep time.

Even humans appear to have more than one way to receive information about light and dark. While the eyes serve as the primary entryway, recent studies indicate that information about light might also reach the brain through sensors located on skin cells or perhaps in the blood. In fact, a new study by Scott Campbell at Cornell University found that shining a bright light on the back of the knees (a highly vascular area) can reset the biological clock. By applying lights to the knees for three hours during the night, the researchers caused the participants' biological clocks to shift back or forward by a few hours. As we'll show you in Chapter 11, any light of sufficient intensity can cause your body clock to move forward or backward, depending on when you are exposed to it.

Night Owl Wisdom

Entrainment is a word used by sleep researchers to describe the process by which internal biological rhythms, particularly sleep/wake cycles, become synchronized with outside stimuli, like the rising and setting of the sun.

Night Owl Wisdom

Zeitgeber is a German term that means "timegiver." In chronobiology, Zeitgeber refers to the specific external influences that synchronize our internal circadian system.

The Power to Choose

Although light is our primary Zeitgeber, and our biological clock is a strong motivator for our physiological activities and behavior, we aren't forced to follow either one. Instead, you're able to override your biological disposition and willfully shift your bedtimes and wake-up times to accommodate changes in your daily schedule, at least on an occasional basis. It isn't always easy to do so, and some people feel the ill effects of such a shift almost immediately. Clearly, however, you aren't forced to go to sleep or wake up at a set time, at least not biologically speaking.

With this freedom to choose your sleep/wake patterns, however, comes the responsibility to understand nature's laws and human limitations. In the modern world, it is rarely too dangerous to be out in the middle of the night, but if you abuse this freedom, you can all too readily disrupt your sleep patterns and become sleep deprived.

Fortunately, you get help in maintaining a fairly consistent schedule despite your personal, internal clock, not only from the light/dark Zeitgeber, but from a host of other timegivers as well. The timing of meals, the regularly scheduled exercise routine, and the social schedules imposed by work, family, and friends, all of these familiar activities provide a sense of time that keeps the biological clock's pendulum swinging in the appropriate rhythm.

As synchronized as our biological and social Zeitgebers keep us as a society, however, a wide variety of individual differences in rhythms exists from one person to the next. Most are barely noticeable, but two groups of people—those who consistently crave the morning light and those who love to burn the midnight oil—illustrate just how much of a difference the biological clock can make on the way we feel every day.

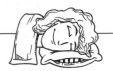

Sleep on it

Don't be lazy if you're having trouble sleeping! Studies show that keeping to a regular exercise routine—that means exercising at about the same time every day or every other day—helps alleviate mild sleep-related circadian rhythm disturbances. (We'll talk more about exercise and sleep in Chapter 13.)

The Larks vs. the Owls

"It's a sin to go to bed the same day you get up," former New York mayor Jimmy Walker once uttered, no doubt enjoying the city's infamous nightlife. The 17th-century philosopher René Descartes claimed he owed his renowned intellect to the fact that he never got out of bed before noon. Both Walker and Descartes were "night owls," and like the bird they emulated, they felt their best in the hours after noon and into the night. Benjamin Franklin, on the other hand, was a lark, rising with—and basking in—the sun. "Early to bed, early to rise makes a man healthy, wealthy, and wise," he wrote, giving the larks of the world an adage to live by.

As you might have guessed, larks and owls have a different cycle in their circadian rhythms, with the owls peaking about 2 hours later than their lark counterparts. This difference occurs in all the physical rhythms, including the daily rise and fall of body temperature and the increase and decrease in hormone levels.

Psychologically, the difference in rhythms is even greater than this biological shift indicates. True larks adore the morning—breakfast tends to be their favorite meal of the day—they are alert and creative early in the day, and they usually spend quiet evenings before going to bed on the early side. Owls, on the other hand, often spurn breakfast (though they usually require caffeine to get them up and running) and only truly blossom as the day progresses. Needless to say, such strong preferences may lead to difficulties with job performance or other responsibilities. A lark who must work the night shift, for instance, is apt to be miserable—and perhaps poor at his or her job. And a night owl might be more than a little cranky if he or she has to drive the morning carpool.

In Chapter 5, you'll take a test that will help you determine whether you have more lark or owl tendencies. Then, in Chapter 8, we'll discuss what happens when a relatively mild lark-owl preference gets out of hand and becomes a true sleep disorder that seriously interferes with daily life. Right now, it's time to learn a little more about what happens to your brain and your body when you do fall asleep. You might be surprised at what happens after "lights out!"

The Least You Need to Know

➤ The human brain contains a cluster of cells that acts as an internal timekeeper and pacemaker.

➤ Many of your daily biological activities and behavior are influenced by internal rhythms.

➤ Your sleep/wake patterns, and how alert you feel at different times of the day, are also regulated by the internal clock.

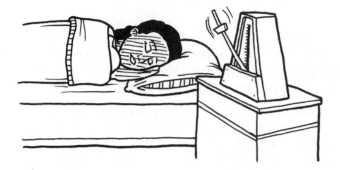

Chapter 3

The Rhythm of the Night

> ## In This Chapter
>
> ➤ The organization of sleep
>
> ➤ From wakefulness to slumber: the stages
>
> ➤ The brain as it dreams
>
> ➤ How sleep restores and refreshes

William Shakespeare once described sleep as "nature's soft nurse," and who among us would argue with him? Nothing feels better after a hard day of living than falling into the sweet oblivion of sleep, then waking up feeling refreshed, renewed, and ready to enjoy the new day.

Despite its restful and restorative qualities, however, sleep is not a static, quiet activity. In fact, a lot happens within the brain while you're getting your nightly shut-eye: Even at the deepest level of sleep, there is only a moderate decrease in brain activity compared to a waking state. If all goes well, you emerge from sleep feeling restored. If something goes wrong, however, you could wake up feeling groggy, cranky, and out of sorts.

What goes on in the brain at night that allows you to get the rest you need? You might just be surprised at how complex your sleep system really is.

The Five Stages of Sleep

"Some must watch while some must sleep/Thus runs the world away."

Shakespeare wrote these lines in *Hamlet* nearly 400 years ago, but he could have been describing the business of a modern 20th-century sleep laboratory. In labs around the world, researchers watch while volunteers sleep. Electrodes attached to volunteers' scalps, faces, and skin record the work going on in their brains and bodies, sketching on a piece of paper or computer screen the physical representation of a night's sleep.

Night Owl Wisdom

A **polysomnograph** is a device used by researchers and physicians to investigate sleep patterns and to help diagnose sleep disorders. It measures brain waves, muscle activity, and eye movements simultaneously. You'll learn more about the polysomnograph in Chapter 5.

Wake Up!

If you consistently wake up in the morning feeling tired and out-of-sorts without knowing why, you may need to see a sleep specialist to track down what really happens as you sleep. Even if you don't remember waking up, something internal or external could be disturbing your sleep without you being aware of it.

As we head toward the new millennium, historians will no doubt comment upon the remarkable advances made in the field of neurobiology—the study of the brain's chemistry and physiology—during the last 40 years or so. The National Institutes of Health even designated the 1990s as "The Decade of the Brain," because research into causes and treatments of such devastating disorders as Huntington's disease, Parkinson's disease, and Alzheimer's disease continued to show great promise.

Nevertheless, scientists would agree that there is still much to learn about the brain and its activities, including what happens during sleep and why. And there's good reason for this lack of knowledge: The technology needed to investigate the hundreds of millions of tiny brain cells and the chemicals that fuel their communication is still being developed. Indeed, when it comes to sleep research in particular, the tools needed to accurately measure brain activity were developed within only the last few decades.

One such device is the *polysomnograph,* a machine that simultaneously measures several different body functions (brain-wave patterns, muscle activity, eye movements, and heart rate). It uses electrodes attached to the scalp to reveal the complex interactions among brain cells. This has helped scientists better understand the "architecture of sleep," or the organization and rhythm of the night.

As mentioned in Chapter 1, sleep has two basic components: a deep non-Rapid Eye Movement (abbreviated NREM) sleep and Rapid Eye Movement (REM) sleep, during which most dreaming occurs. NREM sleep is further divided into four stages of various intensities. These stages recur four or five times during the average 8 hours of sleep, in an orderly progression. Please note, however, that the length of time spent in each stage of sleep, and total sleep time, changes at different stages of life, a fact we'll discuss in more depth in Part 4.

The time from Stage 1 of NREM to the first REM sleep is called the first "sleep cycle," and the time from then to the end of the next REM sleep is the second sleep cycle. There are usually about four or five sleep cycles a night—each lasting about 90 to 100 minutes per cycle. The amount of each sleep stage within a cycle changes throughout the night. In the first half of the night there is more deep sleep (NREM Stages 3 and 4); and in the second half, REM takes over, making up more and more of each sleep cycle. Your final REM phase can last up to 30 minutes or more.

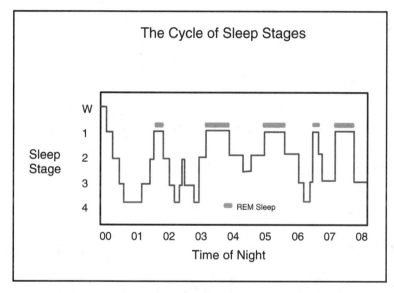

You cycle through the four sleep stages and a period of REM sleep several times each night, with each cycle taking about 90 to 100 minutes.

In later chapters, we'll discuss how these stages and cycles change with age and with various sleep disorders. In the meantime, let's take a look at how the average young adult with a normal, healthy sleep pattern passes the night.

Stage 1: Drowsy Is as Drowsy Does

You know that drowsy feeling that comes over you when you're lying in bed, getting ready to fall asleep? That's Stage 1 sleep. Stage 1 marks the transition from wakefulness to sleep: The world of noise and light begins to fade away as your eyes begin to feel heavy, your muscles relax, your heart rate and breathing slow down and become very steady. The initial bout of Stage 1 sleep usually lasts about 10 minutes and small amounts occur occasionally thereafter. During Stage 1, you may be half aware of the world around you. In fact, if you are awakened out of Stage 1, you may deny that you fell asleep—even though it was perfectly obvious to your partner that you were asleep.

As we become drowsy, a regular pattern (8 to 12 cycles per second) appears in our brain waves called *alpha* waves. Then as we transition into Stage 1 sleep, brain activity slows further as wavy lines of 3 to 8 cycles per second appear, called *theta* waves. Compare this to the "awake" rhythm of rapid fluctuations, and you can appreciate that the brain is slowing down, relaxing, and becoming less aroused by, and aware of, external stimuli.

This figure shows how brain wave patterns change from wakefulness to drowsiness, and then through the 4 stages of non-REM sleep and REM sleep.

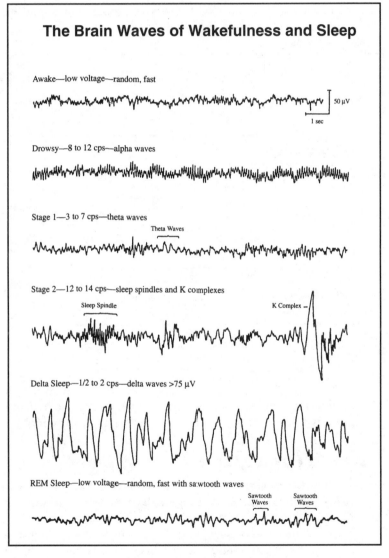

The Brain Waves of Wakefulness and Sleep

Awake—low voltage—random, fast

50 μV

1 sec

Drowsy—8 to 12 cps—alpha waves

Stage 1—3 to 7 cps—theta waves

Theta Waves

Stage 2—12 to 14 cps—sleep spindles and K complexes

Sleep Spindle

K Complex

Delta Sleep—1/2 to 2 cps—delta waves >75 μV

REM Sleep—low voltage—random, fast with sawtooth waves

Sawtooth Waves

Sawtooth Waves

From Hauri, P, The Sleep Disorders *(The Upjohn Company) 1982 with permission.*

Stage 2: Look Who's Asleep Now

Stage 2 is the first true sleep state, but it is still very light sleep.

Stage 2 shows up on the EEG as bursts of activity lasting only a second or two that occur in the context of a background of relatively low-voltage, mixed-frequency activity. These bursts, called *sleep spindles,* sometimes alternate with the *K-complex,* a series of sharp, high-voltage negative waves followed by slow positive waves.

Stages 3 and 4: The Deep

Although Stage 3 and Stage 4 are quite distinct, they are often lumped together as "slow wave sleep." These are the stages in which the body is believed to carry out most of its repair and restoration work. Within about 20 minutes of lying down to sleep, you fall into Stage 3 sleep, the first stage of deep sleep. Your body temperature falls, and your breathing and heart rate slow considerably. Once you're here, you're *really* asleep. If someone tries to wake you, they're apt to have a hard time, and you're likely to feel groggy and disoriented if they succeed. You only spend a few minutes here, however, before falling into the deepest sleep.

On the EEG, brain waves continue to develop into mostly large, slow waves during Stage 3 sleep. Up to 50 percent of brain waves at this stage are slow waves known as "delta" waves.

Night Owl Wisdom

Sleep spindles and **K-complexes** are types of brain waves associated with Stage 2, or light, sleep. They are named for the distinctive, sharp shapes they make on the EEG that represent sporadic brain activity.

Night Owl Wisdom

Stages 3 and 4 are also known as **delta** or "slow wave" sleep after the slow, deep waves they make on the EEG in contrast to the rapid irregular undulations made during wakefulness.

Stage 4 is the deepest level of sleep. During the first cycle of sleep, we arrive at Stage 4 approximately 1 hour after falling into Stage 1 sleep. On the EEG, Stage 4 sleep is represented by high-voltage, slow-frequency delta waves that occur more than 50 percent of the time.

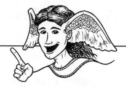

Morpheus Says

Have you ever wondered what that gunk you wipe out of the edges of your eyes in the morning really is? It turns out that when you sleep at night, your eyes still blink and move around (especially during REM sleep when you're dreaming) and tears still move across your eyes to keep them wet and clean. These tears carry small bits of mucus and dust, which tends to collect at either edge of the eye during the night. And that's what you wipe away as you greet the day.

REM: Life Is but a Dream

The final stage of sleep is REM sleep, the phase of sleep in which you dream. Your first bout of REM comes about 90 minutes after the start of sleep. Usually, you'll first rise from a deep NREM Stage 3 or 4 sleep into a light Stage 2 sleep before starting the first REM phase. REM sleep is markedly different physiologically from NREM sleep: Not only is your brain more active, but your blood pressure, heart beat, and respiration rates may rise as well.

As you can see in the previous figure, EEG brain wave readings reveal that REM sleep looks almost identical to wakefulness, which shows you how hard your brain is working while you're dreaming. The characteristic rapid eye movements and the lack of muscular activity that show up on the polysomnograph, however, make it clear what's actually happening.

Now that you have some idea of the stages of sleep, you might be wondering what scientists think is really going on as you climb up and down the staircase of consciousness, sleep, and dreaming.

The Dream of REM

REM sleep is also known as "paradoxical" sleep, and for good reason. First, the brain is working so hard that it's almost like being awake. Second, the brain is very active but the body is motionless. As mentioned in Chapter 1, a nerve center in the brain keeps muscles in a state of near paralysis during REM sleep. If this did not occur, you'd be acting out your dreams while still unconscious.

For centuries, artists and philosophers have pondered the meaning of dreams; and more recently, scientists and physicians have searched for the medical purpose and consequences of dreams. An important step along the way took place in 1953, when a young researcher named Nathaniel Kleitmann noticed that the eyes of his sleeping 8-year-old son periodically moved about, back and forth, as if he were watching a silent movie inside of his head. Digging out an old EEG machine from the basement of the University of Chicago where he studied, Kleitmann recorded his son's brain waves while he slept. The readings revealed a brain so active it might as well have been awake. He and his colleagues named this sleep "Rapid Eye Movement" sleep, or REM sleep.

Suspecting a connection between REM sleep and dreaming, Kleitmann, sleep pioneer William C. Dement, and other researchers set about proving that theory the only way possible: In study after study, they woke people out of REM sleep and asked them about their dreams. The answers confirmed it: Between 80 and 95 percent of REM sleepers reported vivid dreams, compared to only 7 percent of those woken from NREM sleep. (Yes, you do occasionally dream while in other sleep stages, but the primary dream stage is REM sleep.)

During REM sleep, then, we're awake within ourselves, thinking and performing in an altered state. In Chapter 23, we'll discuss what philosophers, psychiatrists, and artists believe dreams represent to our minds and souls. In addition to the metaphysical meaning of dreams, however, REM sleep apparently serves a biological purpose. What the purpose is, and why it developed, on the other hand, remain questions in need of answers.

One theory is that REM sleep helps consolidate memory and emotion. We know, for instance, that blood flow during REM sleep rises sharply in several brain areas linked to the processing of memories and emotional experiences. Blood flow declines, on the other hand, in areas involved in complex reasoning and language located at the front of the brain.

Sleep studies performed at the Weizmann Institute in Israel seem to confirm this theory. Subjects were shown various objects on a computer screen and then tested later for recall. After depriving some of the subjects of REM sleep, researchers found that memory recall was impaired in that group, while the subjects who slept uninterrupted had no changes in performance.

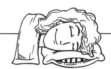

Sleep on it

Time your naps. If you need to get rid of your drowsiness, for best results, take a 15- or 20-minute nap—just long enough to reach Stage 2 sleep, but not long enough to reach the deepest sleep. A nap of this length will suffice if you're pressed for time, but if you can afford it, nap for about 90 minutes, which will take you through one whole sleep cycle. That way, you might even get in an interesting dream!

Night Owl Wisdom

A **neurotransmitter** is a chemical that allows nerve cells to communicate with one another and with other cells in the body.

Other studies supporting the memory consolidation connection suggest the involvement of the *neurotransmitter* called acetylcholine in the process. Known for its role in the process of memory (it is produced by the same brain cells damaged in memory disorders like Alzheimer's disease) and found throughout the body, acetylcholine levels surge during REM sleep, but not in other sleep stages.

In any case, the need for REM sleep is certain: If deprived of it for one or more nights, you'll wake up feeling irritable and unable to concentrate. Then you'll "reimburse" yourself by dreaming more the next time you get a full night's sleep. In fact, on the following nights, your dreaming will start sooner and last much longer, consuming a greater percentage of total sleep time than usual.

The same can be said for the other stages of sleep, collectively known as NREM. As much as we need to dream, we also need to heal and to restore. If deprived of Stages 3 and 4 sleep, you'll wake up feeling extremely sleepy the next day, no matter how much light sleep and REM sleep you've enjoyed.

The Depth of Non-REM

Your body is relaxed, your brain is at rest, and you're able to move around a bit to get more comfortable without waking up: Now this is what sleep is *really* supposed to be like, isn't it? NREM sleep, which accounts for about 80 percent of the total sleep time of the average young adult, appears to restore the body in the same way that REM sleep may help restore the brain and the emotions.

First, and perhaps most important, the body truly rests during NREM sleep. All physiological functions—body temperature, blood pressure, heart rate, respiration rate, digestion, urinary function, and brain activity—slow down. Although you're able to move about (the average person shifts body position more than 30 times a night), muscles are relaxed. Interestingly enough, studies indicate that our muscles might receive just as much relaxation and repair during simple rest periods, and that the state of unconsciousness we call sleep may not be necessary for this purpose. It seems that our brains need sleep far more than our bodies do—no matter how good it feels to hit the sheets after a hard day of physical work and play!

In addition, your body produces a much-needed hormone during sleep—one that helps repair and maintain your muscles and bones. During Stages 3 and 4 of NREM sleep, the body receives almost all of its daily dose of an important hormone called *human growth hormone* (HGH). HGH is secreted by the pituitary, an endocrine gland located at the base of the brain. A protein hormone, HGH promotes the growth, maintenance, and repair of muscles and bones by facilitating the use of

Night Owl Wisdom

Human growth hormone (HGH) is secreted by the pituitary gland and works to promote the growth and repair of the body. Without NREM sleep, HGH is not released to do its work.

amino acids, the essential building blocks of protein. Although the actual synthesis of protein and repair of muscles may take place both during the day and at night, the body does require NREM sleep in order to release the hormone in the first place.

In the end, then, it's clear that both main phases of sleep—REM and NREM—are necessary for the maintenance of good health and good cheer.

A Good Night's Sleep

Allan Hobson, one of the leading neurobiologists studying sleep today, wrote, "Nature is much too economical to waste hours of biological time doing nothing but simply saving energy and idling the brain….A night of sleep is as much preparation for the subsequent day's activity as recovery from that of the previous day."

Without question, sleep is as important to your health as proper nutrition and regular exercise—and quality of sleep appears to be just as important as quantity. Indeed, even if you sleep for 8 or 9 hours, you may still suffer from the effects of too little sleep if you spend too much time in the lighter stages of sleep and not enough in the deeper stages and REM periods. Or perhaps you suffer from one of the many sleep disorders, such as sleep apnea or Restless Leg Syndrome (discussed in Chapter 5), that disrupt you—and your partner perhaps—without your being aware of the problem. In some cases, you might be able to track down the culprit yourself, using the tips we give you in the coming chapters. In other cases, you may need the help of a qualified professional trained in the fine art of sleep research.

If you're not getting a good night's sleep, you're not alone. Millions of Americans do not get enough quality sleep and thus suffer the effects of sleep deprivation. In the next chapter, we'll show you how dangerous and downright debilitating sleep deprivation can be.

The Least You Need to Know

➤ The brain works very hard during sleep.

➤ REM sleep, or dreaming sleep, helps consolidate your memories and emotions.

➤ Quality of sleep is just as important as quantity of sleep when it comes to good health and feelings of well-being.

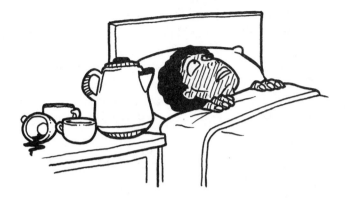

Chapter 4

It's Not as Easy as It Looks

In This Chapter

➤ Exploring the medical causes of sleep problems

➤ Identifying a sleep disorder

➤ Focusing in on bad habits and lifestyle issues

At this point on your journey toward a good night's sleep, you've reached a fork in the road: One avenue leads to what we call "normal" sleep problems caused mainly by lifestyle habits and situations; and the other leads to "pathological" sleep problems, caused by medical conditions or medications. In this chapter, we help you determine which fork in the road you should take first.

Eating a balanced diet, exercising on a regular basis, reducing stress, sleeping well: Most of us know the prescription for a long and healthy life, but few of us actually follow it. More than 60 million Americans have difficulty with sleep, and more than 35 percent of us are now officially overweight. Heart disease—much of it related to an anxiety-ridden, energy-sapping, sleep-disrupting lifestyle—remains our number one killer. Of non-disease–related deaths, traffic accidents head the list, and many of them can be blamed directly or indirectly on sleep deprivation. Indeed, at least two studies, one by the Oklahoma Turnpike Authority and one by the California Division of Highways, suggest that as many as 50 percent of the fatal accidents on freeways are caused by drivers falling asleep or briefly nodding off.

All together, the typical late 20th-century lifestyle is proving to be detrimental to your health and to your sleep. Both the body and the mind suffer if you do not get the sleep you need, and that's something far too few of us take seriously.

On the other hand, it's important not to start blaming the victim (namely, you in this case!) for his or her own sleep problem. You're up against a huge array of social, economic, and technological imperatives that drive you to neglect your health (including your sleep needs) in all kinds of ways.

In addition, a sleep problem can become chronic and debilitating before you know it. Once you have a night or two of poor sleep, you start dragging through the day, eating poorly and exercising less; you become anxious about sleep as the night wears on, then toss and turn despite your exhaustion. You suffer, silently or not so silently, for weeks, even years before figuring out how to solve your problem.

Now, however, you've taken the proverbial bull by the horns by reading this book. So far, you've learned a great deal about your own internal clock and how it sets your rhythms, and about your own sleep patterns. In this chapter, we'll show you the wide variety of medical conditions and specific sleep disorders that can cause a sleep problem, and we give you advice about when to seek help from a medical professional.

Tracking Down the Culprit

Drinking too much caffeine. Asthma. Snoring. Nightmares. Heart disease. Medications. Depression. Rich foods consumed too late at night. Alcohol consumption before bedtime. Arthritis. Stress. An uncomfortable mattress or pillow.

We could go on and on. Indeed, the list of potential sleep disrupters is a pretty long one, which is what may make it difficult to diagnose a sleep problem, not only for a regular person like yourself but also for medical doctors and sleep specialists. In most cases of mild to moderate sleep difficulties, lifestyle issues—including time zone travel, shift work, diet and exercise habits, and stress levels—are the likely culprits, and the exploration of those subjects form the core of this book.

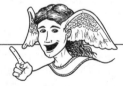

Morpheus Says

You might be surprised at how long one person can manage to stay awake if he puts his mind to it: Randy Gardner managed to survive after staying awake for 264 hours—11 entire days—and 12 minutes in 1965, setting a world's record that no one's beaten yet. (For the record, Randy then slept for 14 hours and 40 minutes straight, a relatively small amount of time when you consider how long he'd been up.)

For now, though, we want to stress that if you have a stubborn sleep problem and haven't had a recent check-up with your primary physician, now is the time to make that appointment. There are a host of medical problems that could be keeping you up at night, and it's important to rule out those conditions first. In fact, here are the general categories that medical professionals consider when attempting to zero in on the cause of a particular sleep problem:

➤ medical conditions

➤ psychiatric problems

➤ sleep disorders

Some doctors may start with the medical and work their way down the list, while others may focus on what they consider the most likely culprit based on your medical and personal history. Let's take these issues one by one.

The Body Connection

Chronic pain, heart disease, stomach ulcers, and many other medical illnesses can disrupt your sleep by increasing the amount of time it takes to fall asleep, by increasing the number of times you wake up, and by decreasing the overall depth of sleep throughout the night.

The good news is that once the underlying problem is identified and treated, the sleep problem often dissipates as well. The bad news is that certain medications designed to treat these very same conditions could end up upsetting your sleep. That's why it's essential that you talk with your doctor about your sleep patterns, along with any other medical symptoms you experience, on a regular basis.

Clearly, it goes far beyond the scope of this book to explore the full range of sleep-related medical issues. What we'll do, however, is give you a list of the most common medical conditions affecting sleep so that you can discuss them with your doctor.

➤ *Arthritis*. Arthritis is a general term for more than 100 different conditions that cause inflammation—and usually swelling and pain—of the joints. In all forms of arthritis, the pain often becomes worse at night, which increases the time spent awake in bed and the amount of light sleep during the night. Unfortunately, a vicious circle often ensues, since the stress of insomnia often worsens the course of some forms of arthritis.

➤ *Headaches*. Headaches come in many forms and have many different causes. There are the throbbing migraines, the aching sinus headaches, the run-of-the-mill tension headaches, and a host of others. Most of the time, headaches are not life threatening and will pass on their own or with the aid of analgesics or other medication. If you have severe headaches that disturb your sleep, however, it's important to see your doctor for an evaluation.

➤ *Frequent urination.* Any condition that sends you to the bathroom several times a night—a condition called *nocturia*—will disrupt your sleep. Urinary tract infections are a common problem for women of all ages, and the risk more than triples over the age of 60. Also more common among older women is urinary incontinence. Among men, the most common cause of frequent urination is an enlarged prostate gland, which affects about 75 percent of men over age 50. For most people, the return to sleep is rapid, but for those who can't fall back to sleep quickly, a sleep debt accumulates rapidly. If you feel that you wake up because you need to urinate, talk to you doctor no matter what your age.

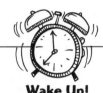

Wake Up!

Don't assume that a need to urinate is what actually wakes you up during the night. A 1997 study in the *Journal of the American Medical Association* showed that other sleep problems, particularly sleep apnea, caused the initial awakening in a group of older adults, who only then felt the need to urinate. Talk to your doctor if you have this problem.

➤ *Breathing problems.* It stands to reason that any medical condition that interferes with breathing would disrupt sleep. Such conditions include asthma, emphysema and other chronic lung conditions, and allergies. They often result in increased wakefulness and more time spent in lighter sleep.

➤ *Heart disease.* Any form of heart disease, including angina (severe chest pain that occurs when the oxygen supply to the heart is interrupted), arrhythmias (disturbed heart rhythms), coronary artery disease, and congestive heart disease can cause sleep problems. In addition, the medication used to treat these conditions can also disturb sleep. Some may also trigger chronic nightmares.

➤ *Stomach problems.* Difficulty getting to sleep, fragmented sleep, frequent awakenings...you name it, and a gastrointestinal tract problem can cause it. In peptic ulcer disease, lesions develop in the stomach, causing a dull pain to occur about 1 to 4 hours into the night. The pain can radiate into the chest or back and be accompanied by a burning sensation in the stomach or chest and a feeling of fullness, nausea, or cramping. Gastroesophageal reflux—also known as heartburn—is another common problem in which stomach fluid or contents from the stomach are regurgitated into the esophagus during sleep. In most cases reflux doesn't lead to full awakening, but some sleepers wake up coughing or choking, with a sour taste in the mouth, burning at the back of the throat, and pain in the stomach or chest.

➤ *Allergies.* Who could sleep with an itchy rash, a raspy cough, or a headache caused by stuffed sinuses? All of these allergy-related symptoms, and others, can disrupt sleep patterns—and so can the drugs used to treat them.

➤ *Nervous system disorders.* Any condition that involves a disruption of brain chemistry can also disrupt sleep, including Parkinson's disease, epilepsy, muscular dystrophy, Tourette's syndrome, Huntington's chorea, dystonia, and others. These conditions increase the number of awakenings, shifts between the stages of sleep, and the amount of time spent in light rather than deep sleep. And as is true for so many other medical conditions, the medications used to treat nervous system disorders may also disturb sleep.

➤ *Menstruation, pregnancy, and menopause.* As we'll discuss in depth in Chapter 21, thanks to the hormone fluctuations they experience, women have special problems with sleep. Changing hormone levels during the week before menstruation, for instance, can increase the time it takes to go to sleep or can cause multiple awakenings. Pregnant women tend to crave a lot more sleep than usual, especially during the first three months. Conversely, weight gain, bloating, and the presence of a six- or eight-pound fetus during the last three months of pregnancy make it difficult to get to and stay asleep. The drastic decrease in estrogen levels during menopause cause a host of symptoms that can interfere with sleep, especially *hot flashes* with their excessive sweating and increase in heart rate.

Night Owl Wisdom

A **hot flash** is the most common symptom of menopause, suffered by at least 75 percent of menopausal women. It generally involves a sudden rush of heat to the upper body that starts in the chest area and spreads to the arms, neck, and face. It can last anywhere from 3 to 5 minutes each and is a harmless—if uncomfortable—reaction to a hormonal imbalance.

The Mind and Sleep Patterns

Although we tend to put psychiatric problems into a different medical "basket" from physical illnesses, it really is impossible to separate the two. Every day, we gain new insight into the immutable mind-body connection—and nowhere is this connection more evident than with sleep problems. In addition to affecting your mood, most psychiatric problems are essentially medical conditions, with physical causes and symptoms that almost always affect sleep patterns. Two of the most commonly diagnosed mood disorders are depression and anxiety.

➤ *Depression.* According to the National Institute of Mental Health, more than 1 in 20 Americans—some 17.8 million people—suffer from depression every year. Along with overwhelming feelings of despair, worthlessness, and guilt, depression also causes physical symptoms that include weight loss or weight gain, gastrointestinal problems, and changes in sleep patterns. Usually people with depression suffer from very early morning awakenings—that's why F. Scott Fitzgerald, who suffered from depression himself, once wrote, "In a real dark night of the soul, it is always three o'clock in the morning, day after day." But sometimes people with depression also have trouble getting to sleep.

People with Seasonal Affective Disorder (SAD), a type of depression that usually occurs in the fall and winter months when day lengths are shorter, tend to sleep too much because they lack exposure to sufficient bright light. According to the

Diagnostic and Statistical Manual of Mental Disorders, 40 to 60 percent of outpatients with major depression and up to 90 percent of hospitalized depressed patients suffer from sleep problems.

➤ *Anxiety disorders.* At any given time, 10 to 15 million Americans suffer the debilitating symptoms of an anxiety disorder, and of this number, three-fourths report a sleep disturbance. Usually, people with anxiety have trouble falling and then staying asleep, and experience fragmented and unrefreshing sleep.

Medication

Ever hear the expression "sometimes the cure is worse than the disease"? Well, it certainly holds true when it comes to medical illnesses and sleep problems. A whole host of drugs used to treat a very wide range of medical and psychiatric conditions can make it difficult for you to sleep well. At the same time, there are medications that actually promote sleep, or at least make you sleepy; but too often, these effects occur at the wrong time (like while you're driving or trying to concentrate). We list the following medications according to their likely effect on your sleep patterns. If you take any of these medications and find you're having trouble sleeping during the night or staying awake during the day, discuss the matter with your doctor. There may well be another, equally effective drug that will not cause this debilitating side effect.

➤ amphetamines—act as stimulants

➤ antidepressants—act as both sedatives and stimulants

➤ antihypertensives—act as both sedatives and stimulants

➤ antihistamines—act as sedatives

➤ appetite suppressants—act as stimulants

➤ benzodiazapines—act as sedatives

➤ corticosteroids—act as stimulants

➤ estrogen replacement—acts as a stimulant

➤ levodopa—acts as a sedative

➤ theophylline—acts as a stimulant

➤ thyroid hormones—act as sedatives

The Sleep Disorders

In addition to the medical conditions and types of medication that indirectly cause sleep problems, there are several disorders directly related to sleep—and millions of Americans suffer from one or more of them without being aware of it. In fact, the National Commission on Sleep Disorders Research estimates that 95 percent of people with sleep disorders are undiagnosed and untreated.

If you're one of them, your problem may warrant a visit to a sleep lab (see Appendix A for more information about where to find a sleep laboratory near you). There, sleep specialists will run a series of tests to determine the underlying cause. Depending on your symptoms, your tests might involve one or more of the following:

➤ *Polysomnography.* As described in Chapter 1, the polysomnograph measures brain wave patterns, muscle activity, eye movements, and heart rate while a subject sleeps (or tries to!). These measurements will help sleep specialists determine how much of each stage of sleep you obtain, how often and how long you dream, and how many times you awaken during the night. By doing so, they can often identify the cause of your sleep problem, and help you find ways to improve it.

➤ *Sleep and breathing tests.* In order to determine whether or not a respiratory problem might be causing a sleep problem such as Obstructive Sleep Apnea, sleep specialists measure breathing patterns, blood oxygen levels, and respiration rates.

➤ *Multiple Sleep Latency Test.* In some cases, a night in a sleep lab is sometimes followed by a day-long examination of your daytime alertness levels. The test— called MSLT for short—helps determine how sleepy you are during the day by timing how long it takes you to fall asleep during times when you'd usually be awake. Every 2 hours, you'll be asked to try to fall asleep, and lab personnel measure the time it takes you to nod off. If you fall asleep in less than 5 minutes, you may well suffer from a sleep disorder. If you don't have a sleep problem, you'll probably take about 10 to 20 minutes to fall asleep.

In any case, you should talk to your doctor about seeking the help of a sleep specialist if your sleep problems are particularly stubborn or if, after reading the next several sections, you think you may be suffering from a sleep disorder.

Loud and Not So Clear

Snoring and Obstructive Sleep Apnea are two different, but often related, conditions that can interfere with proper sleep. Take the following quiz to see if you might be affected by one or both of them.

1. I know or have been told that I snore loudly.
   True _____ False _____

2. I often wake up feeling short of breath.
   True _____ False _____

3. My partner has heard me gasping for breath, or heard me stop breathing for more than a few seconds while asleep.
   True _____ False _____

If you've answered true to the first question, you already know who you are—a snorer! If you've been having trouble sleeping, or don't feel rested during the day, your snoring may be waking you up or keeping you from sleeping deeply. Your partner (if you have one) may also be suffering because the noise of your snoring keeps him or her up at night.

Night Owl Wisdom

Obstructive Sleep Apnea is a physical disorder in which normal breathing patterns are interrupted because your airways collapse during sleep. When your body recognizes that it isn't getting the oxygen it needs, you abruptly wake up, disturbing the orderly progression of the normal sleep cycle.

A true answer to questions 2 and 3, especially if you've also answered "true" to the first question, strongly indicates that you suffer from a related disorder called Obstructive Sleep Apnea. In sleep apnea, your airways collapse, which causes periodic reductions or complete interruptions in airflow during sleep. In other words, you stop breathing while you are asleep until the brain finally gets the message that the body needs more oxygen. At that point, you wake up, usually snorting and gasping for air, and most of the time not realizing that you're doing so. You drift back to sleep quickly, and the problem starts all over again—in fact, it can happen hundreds of times a night. A person with sleep apnea tends to get lots of Stage 1 sleep (the lightest) at the expense of the deeper, more restorative Stages 3 and 4 and REM sleep. If you think your snoring has become a problem, or that you suffer from sleep apnea, read Chapter 7 with care and seek the advice of your doctor.

Up in the Night

As you may remember from Chapter 1, lying flat and in relative stillness are two hallmarks of sleep. Millions of Americans, however, move about freely—far too freely—during the night, preventing themselves and often their partners from getting a good night's sleep. See if you're one of them by answering the following questions:

1. I often experience a "creepy crawly" feeling or other unusual sensation in my lower legs in the evening before I go to sleep or just after I wake up.
   True _____ False _____

2. I often have to get out of bed or shake my leg to relieve pain or discomfort.
   True _____ False _____

3. I've been told that I twitch or jerk a lot when I'm asleep.
   True _____ False _____

Copyright © 1998 by Circadian Information Limited Partnership. Reprinted with permission. All rights reserved.

If you answer true to questions 1 and 2, you may be suffering from a condition called *Restless Leg Syndrome* (RLS). If question 3 sounds like you, you may have a related condition, called *Periodic Limb Movement Disorder*. These conditions cause unpleasant or painful sensations like tickling, deep aching, or mild to severe muscle spasm in the lower limbs. The pain occurs most often just before sleep but also may occur during the sleep period. Stretching, flexing, or repositioning the limb—even getting up and walking—is the only way to get relief. Needless to say, this can upset both your own and your partner's sleep. EEG readings show that these twitches and movements cause arousal in the brain that increases light sleep and decreases deeper stages.

Weirdness After Dark

You probably won't be surprised to learn that certain abnormal behaviors, such as sleepwalking, bed-wetting, and acting out one's dreams (a condition called REM Behavior Disorder), tend to disrupt sleep. Nightmares and night terrors also upset your ability to get the sleep you need. Answer these questions to find out if you suffer from an abnormal sleep behavior, also known as a *parasomnia*.

> **Night Owl Wisdom**
>
> A **parasomnia** is any behavioral disturbance that occurs during sleep, such as bedwetting, sleep walking or talking.

1. I've been told that I frequently talk in my sleep.
   True _____   False _____

2. I walk in my sleep.
   True _____   False _____

3. I've woken up to find that I've eaten food while I thought I was asleep.
   True _____   False _____

4. I wet the bed.
   True _____   False _____

5. I suffer from nightmares or night terrors.
   True _____   False _____

6. I often awaken feeling confused.
   True _____   False _____

Copyright © 1998 by Circadian Information Limited Partnership. Reprinted with permission. All rights reserved.

If you've answered true to any of these questions, you may be suffering from a behavioral sleep disturbance. In Chapter 11 we'll discuss both Restless Leg Syndrome and the parasomnias in depth and provide you with some tips that will help you help control these behaviors. Like other sleep disorders, however, solving such problems often requires help from medical specialists.

The Mistimed Clock

Remember the information we gave you in Chapter 2 about internal body rhythms? Needless to say, if you're trying to sleep when your body wants to stay up, or vice versa, you're going to run into trouble. See if such a situation applies to you by answering true or false to the following statements:

1. I work a night shift or rotating shift.
   True _____   False _____

2. I tend to fall asleep much later than I want to.
   True _____   False _____

3. I regularly fall asleep much earlier than I want to.
   True _____ False _____

4. On weekends and vacations, I go to bed and wake up at significantly different times than I do on my regular schedule.
   True _____ False _____

5. Even on a regular work schedule, I am unable to keep a consistent sleep schedule no matter how hard I try.
   True _____ False _____

If you've answered true to two or more of these statements, you may be suffering from a circadian rhythm disorder. If so, you'd probably be able to get enough sleep, if only you could sleep when your body prefers to. In Chapters 8, 9, and 10, we'll help you make the best of your particular circadian rhythm problem, as well as identify when you might need the help of a sleep specialist.

Lifestyle Issues 101

Thought you were going to get away scot-free, didn't you? Maybe it's a medical problem, you're thinking, or my internal clock is just out of whack. I'll just go see my doctor or a sleep specialist and we'll straighten the whole thing out. While that may be true, you still need to take a look at the way your own daily habits or personal situation may be affecting your sleep, or lack of it. Answer true or false to the following statements:

1. I exercise every evening, an hour before I go to sleep.
   True _____ False _____

2. I never exercise.
   True _____ False _____

3. I drink caffeinated beverages every day, even in the evening.
   True _____ False _____

4. I go to bed at different times during the week and on the weekend, depending on my schedule.
   True _____ False _____

5. I feel constantly under personal or professional pressure, and haven't found effective ways to reduce or relieve my stress levels.
   True _____ False _____

6. I've recently suffered a personal loss or trauma.
   True _____ False _____

7. I usually try to fall asleep while watching television.
   True _____ False _____

8. I often need a prescription or over-the-counter medication to help me sleep.
   True _____ False _____

9. I rarely get outside into the daylight.
   True _____ False _____

10. I sleep during the day at odd times.
    True _____ False _____

How many of these statements ring true for you? If you've answered even two or three of them in the affirmative, your daily pattern of activities may need to change in order for you to sleep well. In Part 2 we'll show you just how to do that. Then, in Part 3, we'll explore situations that can disrupt your sleep patterns, such as working the night shift and flying across time zones, and describe the most common sleep disorders, such as snoring and sleep apnea and the parasomnias. You might find it interesting to read through each chapter, but feel free to skip ahead to the chapter covering the problem you think most applies to you and your sleep profile.

The Least You Need to Know

➤ A wide variety of medical conditions and medications can cause sleep problems.

➤ You may not be aware that you have a sleep disorder like Obstructive Sleep Apnea or Restless Leg Syndrome.

➤ Even if you're able to sleep a full 8 hours if left to your own devices, a work or personal schedule that doesn't match your internal rhythms can cause sleep problems.

➤ Every aspect of your daily life—from your diet and exercise habits to how much sunlight you're exposed to—may have an effect on your sleep.

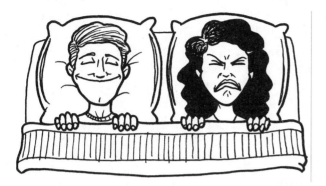

Chapter 5

Your Sleep Personality

> ## In This Chapter
>
> ➤ Exploring your sleep patterns
>
> ➤ Determining your circadian type
>
> ➤ Examining your napping capabilities
>
> ➤ Understanding your sleep personality—and making it work for you

What did you discover about yourself in Chapter 4? Could you have a medical condition or clinical sleep disorder that disrupts your sleep? If so, we certainly hope you'll take our advice and seek help from your doctor and/or a sleep specialist as soon as possible. There's a very good chance that, with the right treatment, you'll soon be sleeping through the night without trouble.

Did you discover, on the other hand, that you're perfectly healthy? While that's certainly very good news, it still leaves you with a sleep problem that has no solution at the moment. The fact is, there are any number of reasons you might be having difficulty with sleep. Some are directly related to your own innate internal biological rhythms. Thus, it is vital that you learn how your particular, highly individual sleep/wake pattern can best be managed.

In this chapter you'll discover your overall "Sleep Personality" by taking a series of quizzes. Your Sleep Personality consists of certain natural tendencies that determine to a large degree when and how well you sleep. First, you'll find out your "Circadian Type"—that is, if you're naturally a morning or a night person. You'll also discover your "Flex-Ability," or how well you can adapt to changes that disrupt your natural rhythms. The next quiz will identify your "Sleep Type"—whether you're a long or short sleeper—by focusing on how much total sleep you need both during your major sleep period (usually occurring at night) and throughout the day (in the form of naps). This aspect of your Sleep Personality relates as well to your napping capability, a trait we'll explore in the quiz about your "Nap-Ability."

You'll also answer some questions having to do with your nighttime responsibilities, such as your work schedule or your need to care for family members during the night. While the first two quizzes focus on your sleep preferences, this one will help you more realistically measure your current chances of sleeping through the night.

Finally, in the section "Are You Getting Enough Sleep?" (Part 2), we'll revisit the question of sleep deprivation to determine if the sleep you get is enough to keep you working and living at an optimal state of alertness and vitality.

We've got a lot to cover, so let's get started.

Night Owl Wisdom

In this book, "Light's Out" refers to the time at which you turn out the light, turn off the TV, and plan to go to sleep. It *does not* refer to the time you get into bed to read or watch the late-night news.

Wake Up!

Be careful not to become addicted to clock-watching during the night. The more concerned you are about what time it is—and how little you've slept—the more anxious you'll become, making it even more difficult for you to fall asleep.

Your Sleep Log

Even before you start answering the questions posed in the quizzes, it's important that you evaluate your current sleep patterns. Frankly, sleep is an activity most of us take for granted, even when we know we could probably get more, or better quality, sleep. To help you more fully understand your own sleep patterns, we've designed a Sleep Log for you to fill in for a week or two—or longer if you work an irregular schedule.

In this log, which appears a little later in this chapter as well as in Appendix C, you'll record several aspects of your sleep life: the time you get into bed, when you turn off the lights (*Lights Out*), the estimated length of time you lay in bed before you actually fall asleep, the estimated number and duration of any awakenings, the time you wake up, the time you get out of bed, and the frequency and duration of naps. To keep a Sleep Log for a week or two, you'll need copies of the log, a pen or pencil to keep by your bed, and an accurate, readable bedside clock.

Just before you turn out the lights, mark down the time. However—and this is important—you should avoid looking at the clock during the night after you check to see what time it is at Lights Out. If you have trouble sleeping—and we'll assume you do since you're reading this book—you shouldn't look at the clock until you're fully awake and ready to roll out of bed in the morning. (We'll talk more about correct "clock etiquette" in Chapter 9.)

Then, when you wake up in the morning, fill out the rest of the log. Try to be as accurate as you can about how long it took you to actually fall asleep after Lights Out, and be sure to make careful note of if and when you woke up during the night and how long it took you to get back to sleep. Another important criterion for you to consider is your *sleep quality*. How do you think you slept? Did you stay awake for a long period of time, anxious and distressed? Did you toss and turn? Wake up constantly? Were you exhausted in the morning? You may find it helpful to rate your *sleep quality* on a scale of one to six, with one being terrible and six being excellent.

You'll also want to track how many hours each day you work—outside or inside the home—and how many hours are spent simply relaxing, as well as how often and for how long you nap during the day. This will help you calculate how much total sleep you need in any 24-hour period, and when your need for a nap occurs most often. We offer you one form here, and another week's worth in Appendix C.

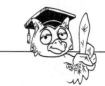

Night Owl Wisdom

Sleep quality refers to your subjective experience of your night's sleep and how it left you feeling. Did you toss and turn? Did you wake up many times or too early in the morning? Did you feel groggy and unsatisfied at wake-up time?

Your Sleep Log

Date _____

Worktime _____

Playtime _____

Bedtime _____

Lights Out _____

Sleep Onset _____

Awakenings:

Number/Length _____

Wake-Up Time _____

Rise Time _____

Sleep Quality (1 = terrible, 2 = poor, 3 = fair, 4 = good,
5 = very good, 6 = excellent) _____

Nap Time/Duration _____

Once you've filled in this log for a week or two, you can start filling in a graph as well. This graph will become a visual representation of your sleep/wake patterns. The following figures show you two different graphs. "The Sleep/Wake Graph of a 9–5 Worker" shows you how the patterns of the "average" person play out, and "The Sleep/Wake Graph of a Shift Worker" illustrates a different kind of pattern.

This graph represents the sleep/wake/activity patterns of a typical person working a 9–5 schedule. During the work week, he gets up between 6 and 7 a.m., works until about 5 or 6 p.m., and goes to bed between 11 p.m. and midnight—which means he sleeps only about 6 or 7 hours per night. Over the weekend, he goes to bed and gets up a bit later.

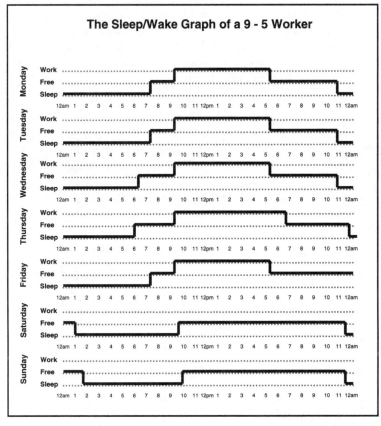

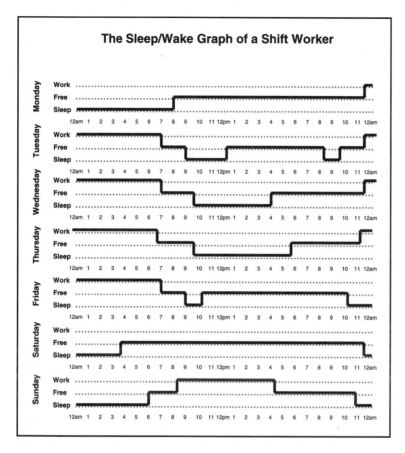

The Sleep/Wake Graph of a Shift Worker

This graph represents the rather nightmarish sleep/wake/activity pattern of a typical shift worker. On Monday, she sleeps until 8 a.m. and then performs chores or has some fun until it's time to go to work at midnight. She works through until 7 a.m., stays up for a bit once she gets home, which means she's been up nearly a full 24 hours straight. Because daytime sleep is difficult even when she is exhausted, she naps for a few hours and then takes another short nap before going to work again at midnight. As you can see, the rest of her week doesn't get a whole lot better; just as she's adjusting to the pattern, she has two days off and loses whatever ground her body clock has gained.

Now, here's a Sleep/Wake Graph for you to fill in, using the data you've collected in your Sleep Log.

You can keep track of your own sleep/wake/activity patterns by filling in this graph for a week.

Your Sleep/Wake Graph

Monday	Work	
	Free	
	Sleep	
		12am 1 2 3 4 5 6 7 8 9 10 11 12pm 1 2 3 4 5 6 7 8 9 10 11 12am
Tuesday	Work	
	Free	
	Sleep	
		12am 1 2 3 4 5 6 7 8 9 10 11 12pm 1 2 3 4 5 6 7 8 9 10 11 12am
Wednesday	Work	
	Free	
	Sleep	
		12am 1 2 3 4 5 6 7 8 9 10 11 12pm 1 2 3 4 5 6 7 8 9 10 11 12am
Thursday	Work	
	Free	
	Sleep	
		12am 1 2 3 4 5 6 7 8 9 10 11 12pm 1 2 3 4 5 6 7 8 9 10 11 12am
Friday	Work	
	Free	
	Sleep	
		12am 1 2 3 4 5 6 7 8 9 10 11 12pm 1 2 3 4 5 6 7 8 9 10 11 12am
Saturday	Work	
	Free	
	Sleep	
		12am 1 2 3 4 5 6 7 8 9 10 11 12pm 1 2 3 4 5 6 7 8 9 10 11 12am
Sunday	Work	
	Free	
	Sleep	
		12am 1 2 3 4 5 6 7 8 9 10 11 12pm 1 2 3 4 5 6 7 8 9 10 11 12am

Whether you use the Sleep Log, the Sleep/Wake Graph, or a combination of both, it's important that you keep careful track of your sleep time. It's also important for you to monitor your schedule on working days, weekends, and—in the best of all possible worlds—during a vacation as well. If you do that, you'll know not only how much you sleep when you have responsibilities that demand your attention but also how much you sleep when you have all the time in the world.

Once you've kept your Sleep Log for a few weeks, you can start to figure out what your natural sleep/wake rhythm is and how much sleep you really need. This rhythm will become even clearer as you take the following quizzes.

Your Circadian and Flex-Ability Profile

The "morning person" (the Lark) is the kind of person who's up with the sun, bustling about, and getting her best work done before lunch. The "night person" (the Owl) is somebody who flourishes in the afternoon and evening and wouldn't care if he never saw the early morning dew again. The intermediate person—who we call the "Regular Robin"—doesn't go to either extreme, but can cope with early mornings and late nights as the need arises.

You know who you are. Or do you? Have you ever really thought about what part of the day truly suits you or when your body would prefer to sleep? We'll help you answer those questions here.

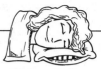

Sleep on it

If you're like most people, your weekends are nearly as busy as your workweek. However, to gain an understanding of your true sleep needs, designate at least one task-free, schedule-free weekend as a "sleep preference" weekend. During this time, sleep—and nap—as much as you want. If, during these periods, you find yourself sleeping significantly more than you normally do, you may be chronically sleep-deprived.

Are You a Lark or an Owl?

This quiz will help sort out the Larks and Owls from the Regular Robins. Consider each question with care and, if need be, check back through your Sleep Log.

Your Circadian Identity

Choose the answer that best relates to your own sleep experience.

1. What time would you get up if you were entirely free to plan your day?
    1 point: Before 7 a.m.
    2 points: 7–9 a.m.
    3 points: After 9 a.m.

2. How easy is it for you to get up on workdays?
    1 point: Fairly easy
    2 points: Moderately difficult/depends on the day
    3 points: Very difficult

3. How alert do you feel during the first 30 minutes after you get up in the morning?
    1 point: Alert/fresh
    2 points: Varies
    3 points: Sleepy/tired

4. What time would you go to bed if it were completely up to you?
    1 point: Before 10:30 p.m.
    2 points: 10:30 p.m.–midnight
    3 points: After midnight

5. How sleepy/tired are you 1¹/₂ hours before going to bed during the workweek?

    1 point: Very tired/ready to fall asleep

    2 points: Moderately tired/depends on the day

    3 points: Not very tired

6. When you've stayed up later than usual (had a late evening), when do you wake up the next morning (assuming you didn't have any alcohol)?

    1 point: At your usual time, with a desire to get out of bed

    2 points: Varies

    3 points: Later than usual, with a desire to fall back asleep

To score this quiz, simply add up your points. You'll come up with a score between 6 and 18. You'll plot this score on the Circadian Type/Flexibility Profile on the following page. Generally speaking, the lower your number, the more of a morning person you are.

How Easygoing Are You?

Are you one of those people who needs to be in bed at the same time every night and has to get your regular amount of sleep or you're just not yourself the next day? Or can you adapt fairly easily to changes in your sleep schedule? Take this quiz to find out.

Your Flex-Ability Quotient

1. When you're feeling drowsy, can you easily overcome it if there is something important you have to do?

    1 point: Rarely

    2 points: Sometimes

    3 points: Usually

2. When you have to do something important in the middle of the night, can you do it almost as easily as you could at a more normal time of the day?

    1 point: Rarely

    2 points: Sometimes

    3 points: Usually

3. Do you enjoy working at unusual times of the day or night?

    1 point: Rarely

    2 points: Sometimes

    3 points: Usually

4. If you have a lot to do, can you stay up late or get up very early to finish it without feeling too tired?

    1 point: Rarely

    2 points: Sometimes

    3 points: Usually

5. Do you find it as easy to work late at night as you do earlier in the day?
   1 point: Rarely
   2 points: Sometimes
   3 points: Usually

6. Do you find it fairly easy to sleep whenever you want to?
   1 point: Rarely
   2 points: Sometimes
   3 points: Usually

Again, total up your score using the point tallies indicated. Generally speaking, the lower your score, the more rigid or inflexible you are about your sleep needs. The higher your score, the more able you are to adapt to outside demands on your time and energy.

Taken together, your scores on these two quizzes place you within a section of the Circadian/Flex-Ability Type Profile that is shown in the following figure. As we've laid it out here, most people fall into one of three general categories: Rigid Lark, Regular Robin, or Flexible Owl.

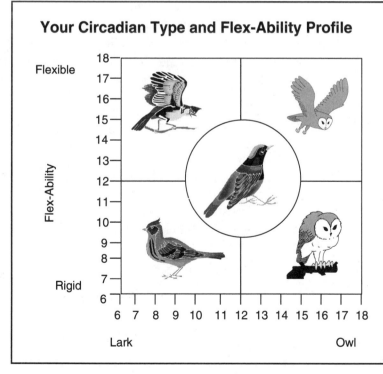

Your Circadian Type and Flex-Ability Profile

Once you've taken the quizzes about your circadian rhythms and your flex-ability, you can plot your scores on this chart. The closer to the middle of the chart the combination of scores brings you, the more of a Regular Robin you tend to be. If you fall into the top half of the chart, you're fairly flexible in your sleep/wake pattern. If you fall into the left side, you have more Lark tendencies, while if your scores place you on the right side, you're more of an Owl.

Night Owl Wisdom

A **Rigid Lark** is someone whose natural sleep pattern gets her up very early in the morning and makes it very difficult for her to sleep in, even if she is forced to stay up past her normal bedtime.

Night Owl Wisdom

Regular Robins have fairly flexible sleep patterns. They generally go to bed before midnight (but not before 10 p.m.), usually wake up after 6 a.m. (but not after, say, 8 a.m.), and adapt fairly easily to changes in this schedule.

Night Owl Wisdom

A **Flexible Owl** is your good old-fashioned "night person" who prefers staying up until after midnight (and maybe even until 1 or 2 a.m.), but but who can adapt to a 9–to–5 routine if need be.

Where did your score put you? If you're someone who rises promptly at 6 a.m. every morning—even when on vacation—and if you have a lot of trouble functioning after your normal bedtime, you're probably in the *"Rigid Lark"* category.

You're a *Regular Robin* if you usually to go to bed between 10 p.m. and midnight, generally wake up between 6 a.m. and 8 a.m., and can manage to function fairly well on either end of the spectrum if circumstances warrant it.

If you're a *Flexible Owl*, you really do crave the night and function best after dinner, but can manage to adjust your regular schedule to keep up with the average 9-to-5 world if necessary.

Here are a few other examples of type-specific behavior and preferences based on these profiles:

If you're a Rigid Lark, you

➤ Would have a hard time staying up late at night, even if you were invited to a Beatles midnight reunion, never mind having to work on your company's annual report

➤ Are a very poor candidate for night-shift work

➤ Might need to learn some special napping strategies if you become sleep-deprived

If you're a Regular Robin, you

➤ May have a preference for working in the morning or evening, but you're not *adamant* about it (like some people!)

➤ Are likely to be rather intolerant of the sleep habits and problems of your Rigid Lark or Flexible Owl counterparts

➤ Can usually follow general prescriptions for getting a good night's sleep

If you're a Flexible Owl, you

➤ Prefer the night, and resist working and playing too early in the morning.

➤ Are an ideal candidate for night-shift work

➤ May get into trouble if you have morning responsibilities but allow yourself to stay up too late at night

As you can see, your natural rhythms have a great deal of influence not only on the way you sleep, but also on how well your body and mind function throughout the day. In the chapters to come, we'll explore how you can use what you know about your Circadian/Flex-Ability Profile to help solve your sleep problems and to help you function better throughout your day and night.

Your Sleep Type and Nap–Ability Profile

The next two quizzes determine how much you want (and probably need) to sleep and how well and how often you nap. Once you determine the answer to those questions, you'll have a greater understanding of what your optimal sleep/wake pattern should be throughout your day.

How Long Is Long Enough?

Some people just love to sleep: 8, 9, even 10 hours of shut-eye a night is perfect for their particular physiological make-up. Other people jump out of bed after what their longer-sleeping counterparts might consider a catnap, but they feel refreshed and rested enough to meet the challenges of the day. To find out which category you fit into, take the following quiz.

Your Sleep Type

Answer each question with one of the following:

1 point: Rarely

2 points: Sometimes

3 points: Usually

1. How many hours of total sleep (night sleep plus daytime naps) of sleep do you usually get per working day? _____

2. How many hours of total sleep do you usually get per day on your days off? _____

3. How many hours of total sleep do you get when you're on vacation? _____

4. How many hours would you sleep when you're not sleep-deprived (when you've just had one or more nights of optimal sleep) and can go to bed and wake up when you want to? _____

5. How many total hours of sleep do you think you need in order to function at your best the next day? _____

Add up your score using the values assigned. Your score will fall between 5 and 40 points, with a score of 5 identifying you as an extremely short sleeper and a score of 40 as an extremely long sleeper. Later, we'll ask you to map this score on the Sleep Type/ Nap-Ability Profile on the following page.

Are You a Napper?

Are you one of those people who can close his eyes for 10 minutes, drift off to dreamland, and then wake up refreshed? Have you made a one- to two-hour siesta a regular part of your day? Or is sleeping during the day difficult—if not impossible—for you? Take this quiz to find out how you score as a napper.

Test Your Nap-Ability

Check your Sleep Log if you need help answering the following questions.

1. Can you easily nap during the daytime when you are not particularly sleep-deprived?
   1 point: Rarely
   2 points: Sometimes
   3 points: Usually

2. Can you easily nap during the daytime to "catch up" on lost sleep, such as after one or more late nights?
   1 point: Rarely
   2 points: Sometimes
   3 points: Usually

3. On days off, do you take a daytime nap?
   1 point: Rarely
   2 points: Sometimes
   3 points: Usually

4. Do you feel refreshed after a daytime nap?
   1 point: Rarely
   2 points: Sometimes
   3 points: Usually

5. Do you use brief naps (less than 30 minutes) to sustain your alertness during an extended monotonous task (for example, driving a long distance) or when staying up all night?
   1 point: Rarely
   2 points: Sometimes
   3 points: Usually

Your total score for this quiz will fall between 5 and 15. The lower your score, the less able you are to nap. The higher your score, the more likely it is that napping forms an integral part of your daily sleep/wake pattern.

Once you find your scores on both of these quizzes, plot the corresponding number on Your Sleep Type and Nap-Ability Profile, shown in the following figure.

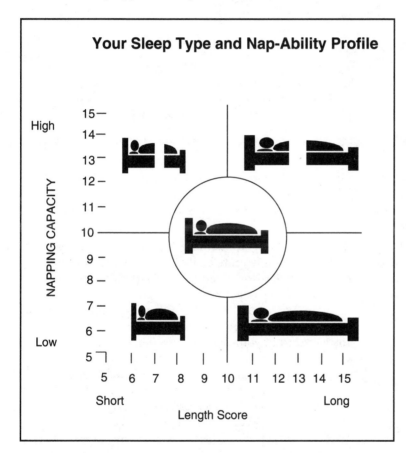

Plot your scores from the Sleep Type and Nap-Ability quizzes on this chart. The closer to the middle of the chart you fall, the more "average" your sleep patterns tend to be—the more likely you are to sleep about 7½ hours a night and nap only occasionally. If your score places you in the top half you like to nap and are able to do so easily—whether you're a short sleeper (on the left side of the chart) or a long sleeper (on the right side of the chart).

Where did your score put you in this profile? Generally speaking, you're in the best shape if you fall into one of these three categories:

➤ *A long sleeper who does not nap.* This means that most of the time you get all the sleep you require during your main sleep period (usually at night). Because you don't nap, you easily become sleep-deprived if something cuts short your main sleep period. This characteristic makes you a less-than-ideal candidate for night-shift work and makes it more likely that you'll suffer from jet lag when you travel.

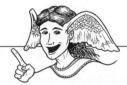

Morpheus Says

A 1997 survey of 802 Cornell University psychology students taken by their professor, James B. Maas, found that more than 80 percent took a nap at least once a week—especially after they learned the importance of getting enough sleep. About 17 percent reported napping at least four days a week; the same percentage said that they never napped.

➤ *An average sleeper who can nap if sleep-deprived.* If you fall into this category, you may need your 6 to 8 hours of sleep (and usually at fairly regular times); but if you miss out on some of them, you can manage to recover by taking a nap at some point during the day.

➤ *A short sleeper who naps.* This means that your main sleep period is relatively short, but you add to your total sleep time quite easily by taking one or more naps during the day. This pattern makes you a perfect candidate for night-shift work and travel across time zones. You can get into trouble, however, if something prevents you from catching up on sleep during the day. You can become sleep-deprived quickly, and displaced from your natural circadian cycle.

Wake Up!

Remember: If a medical condition (arthritis, depression, heart disease, or medication, for example) or a sleep disorder (sleep apnea or a circadian rhythm disorder) is causing your problem, you need to see your doctor or a sleep specialist for advice.

As you can see, each category has its benefits and its risks. Keep in mind that whatever pattern you've developed probably works for you, as long as you're feeling rested and alert during your awake hours, feel that you sleep well, and are able to maintain your work/rest schedule. Just because some sleep experts seem to preach that everyone needs 8 hours doesn't mean that you do.

The only exceptions to this general rule concern those of you who fall outside these three main categories. If you're a very short sleeper—someone who regularly gets less than 5 hours of sleep—who can't nap, for instance, you may well be sleep-deprived because of a clinical sleep disorder or medical problem. The same can be said if you're a very long sleeper—someone who regularly needs more than 9 or 10 hours of sleep—but who still needs to nap during the day on a regular basis. Some underlying medical problem or sleep disorder may be triggering this extreme need for sleep.

No matter how well adjusted you are to your sleep patterns and circadian rhythms, you're apt to be thrown off if you're required to do something important when your body expects to be asleep. The following quiz will help determine if you fall into that category.

Night Work 101

Would you just love to crawl into bed at 11 p.m. and sleep clear through 'til the alarm rings at 6:30—but can't because other responsibilities keep you up all night or drag you from your sleep on a regular basis? If so, you're not alone. Although we tend to think of "night work" as involving factories or all-night diners, many of you may be working through the night for other reasons altogether. Take this quiz to find out.

Your Night Work Evaluation

1. Do you work a fixed night shift?
   Yes _____ No _____

2. Does your work schedule require you to rotate from days to nights on a regular basis?
   Yes _____ No _____

3. Do you routinely work more than 60 hours per week?
   Yes _____ No _____

4. Do you have a family member, such as an infant or ailing parent, who requires your attention during the overnight hours on a regular basis?
   Yes _____ No _____

5. Do you have a second job in addition to your full-time occupation?
   Yes _____ No _____

If you answered yes to one or more of these questions, you should probably go right ahead and read Chapter 15 for information about sleep solutions for your situation. Then, if you're still having trouble, read through the general prescriptions in Part 2 of this book.

That said, it bears repeating that if you wake up feeling rested after spending a peaceful night asleep, your life and your sleep needs are balanced—you're able to sleep when your body craves it, and you wake up having slept enough to function well throughout your day.

If you're reading this book, however, chances are that this is not the case. Something isn't working for you, and you're here to find a solution. The next quiz will help you determine if the sleep you do get—no matter what the circumstances—is enough to sustain you.

Are You Getting Enough Sleep? (Part 2)

In Chapter 1, we asked you to answer several questions about how sleepy you feel during the day so that you would think about your sleep problem in a more concrete way. Here we'll do it again, this time basing our questions on the Epworth Sleepiness Scale, creating a Circadian Technologies version. Your answers will help determine if the sleep you get is enough to sustain you.

On a scale of 0 to 3, rate your likelihood of dozing during the following activities (0 = would never doze; 1 = slight chance of dozing; 2 = moderate chance of dozing; 3 = high chance of dozing):

Activity	Sleepiness Quotient
Sitting and reading	_____
Watching television	_____
Sitting in a lecture or a meeting	_____
As a passenger in a car	_____
Sitting and talking to someone	_____
Driving a car, or stopping for a light	_____
Sitting quietly after lunch	_____

To score this quiz, add up your total. If you score from 0 to 10, congratulations. You are indeed getting enough sleep to keep you awake and alert throughout your day. (However, that doesn't mean you don't have to struggle to get that sleep. If you have trouble falling or staying asleep, it's important that you discover the source of your problem and find a solution, something we can help you do in Part 2.)

If you score from 11 to 15 on this quiz, you need to get more sleep in order to make it through the day safely and with vitality—and you probably know that, which is why you're reading this book! If you score 16 points or more, you're in dire need of more sleep, and chances are you suffer from a serious sleep disorder. We strongly suggest you see your doctor or a sleep specialist as soon as possible to rule out a medical cause.

So Who Are You, Anyway?

What did you learn about your Sleep Personality in this chapter? Did you find out that the way your life is structured coincides with your natural sleep rhythms, or is there a problem in that area? If you've found that you have extreme Lark or Owl tendencies, you may want to skip ahead and read Chapter 16 for some suggestions tailored just for you. Do you need some tips on napping because your nighttime responsibilities interfere with your ability to get enough sleep? Then see Chapter 13.

As you know, many books about sleep fail to consider individual needs and preferences when it comes to discussing solutions to sleep problems and other advice. You'll see that throughout this text, we offer you specific advice targeted to meet the needs of your particular Sleep Personality—and keep your eye out for sidebars titled "Just for You!" in all the chapters that follow.

In the meantime, let's move on to Part 2. For all of you without special problems such as a clinical sleep disorder, nighttime responsibilities, or time-zone travel, this section will help you sleep better, on a schedule that works right for you.

The Least You Need to Know

➤ It's important to become aware of your personal sleep patterns by keeping a Sleep Log.

➤ Determining your Sleep Personality will help you explore your sleep patterns and potential sleep problems with more clarity.

➤ Anyone can become sleep deprived under certain circumstances, and sleep deprivation can undermine your ability to perform your daily responsibilities.

Part 2
Getting a Good Night's Sleep: Your Plan

If you're like most people, the time you choose to start thinking about a solution to your sleep problem is just as you head into your second hour of tossing and turning during the night or just when you're nodding off at an important meeting during the day.

Clearly, neither time represents the best opportunity for coming up with useful, constructive solutions.

Fortunately, a good time has just arrived—right now! In Part 2, we'll show you a variety of ways to increase your chances of getting a good night's sleep—from improving your eating and exercise habits to buying a better mattress and learning how to use light and dark to maintain a sleep/wake cycle that suits your sleep personality.

Read on for a better night's sleep!

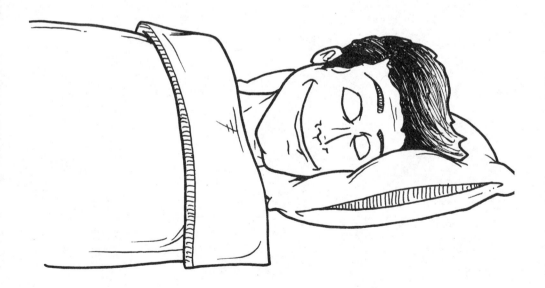

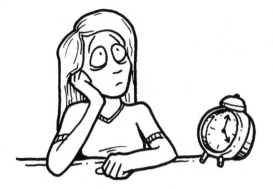

Chapter 6

The World of Sleeplessness

In This Chapter

➤ Insomnia comes in many shapes and sizes

➤ The cause of insomnia may be directly related to your Sleep Personality (Owls vs. Larks, for example)

➤ Sleep deprivation for any reason can cause medical and other problems

➤ Finding a solution to your sleep problems often requires an examination of your daily habits

---

Insomnia—the endless stretch of hours awake in the dark, exhausted, anxious, frustrated. Days spent fighting fatigue in numbing exhaustion. If you're reading this book because you're suffering with insomnia, you know just how physically and emotionally debilitating insomnia can be.

At this point in your journey toward a better night's sleep, we presume you've either ruled out a medical condition or sleep disorder as the cause of your insomnia or received treatment for your condition. In that case, you're here because you still need some help. Or, perhaps, you're a frequent time-zone flyer or shift worker who needs some more advice after reading the chapters that cover your particular situation.

If that's the case, read on. Insomnia is often a treatable condition, one that can be alleviated—if not solved—by making changes in the way you live during the day and in the environment you create for sleep. We discuss those changes in the chapters to come. In the meantime, let's explore the world of insomnia and what it really looks like.

What Kind of Insomniac Are You?

Insomnia isn't one simple condition with just one set of causes, symptoms, and solutions. Some people have trouble sleeping because they drink too much caffeine, others because they exercise too close to bedtime (or not at all), still others because their mattress fails to support their lower back and so they toss and turn in discomfort throughout the night. Emotional upsets, stress overload, and mild illnesses are other possible culprits.

Some people have trouble with falling asleep, others with staying asleep, still others with waking up too early. Many people wake up tired—and then disrupt their normal sleep/wake pattern—because they don't time their sleep properly, thereby interrupting a sleep cycle. (As you may remember from Chapter 3, the brain doesn't like it when you interrupt its REM-NREM cycle at the wrong time!) And then there are the people who have an occasional bad night of sleep, others who have spells of a few weeks or months when sleep is difficult, and still others whose sleep problems become chronic.

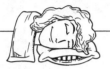

Sleep on it

Be open to a trial-and-error approach to solving your sleep problem. Solving it may require you to evaluate many aspects of your sleeping and waking life, and then making one or more changes until you find yourself sleeping better. For more help, visit our Web site at www.goodsleep.com.

We'll help you sort out some of the reasons you might be having a tough time getting enough sleep later in this chapter with our Bad Sleep Habits Quiz. In the meantime, you may be surprised to learn how very different you may be from your insomniac counterparts, for insomnia does indeed come in all shapes and sizes.

The Basic Types

In considering insomnia from a clinical perspective, sleep specialists categorize three main types: transient, short-term, and chronic. Each type has different qualities and often different solutions:

➤ *Transient insomnia* lasts up to several nights and is often triggered by excitement or stress. Exceptionally good news, or bad, can be so stimulating that sleep becomes difficult, as can extra amounts of exercise too close to bedtime. The first night or two spent away from home, particularly if you've traveled across time zones, can be difficult for sleep. The flu or other brief illnesses can also disrupt normal sleep patterns for a few nights. Transient insomnia usually resolves itself and is no cause for alarm. However, if you become too anxious and worried about not sleeping, you can find yourself caught in a vicious circle that leads to stress-related insomnia: You're so worried about not being able to sleep well, you can't sleep at all. We discuss this problem in more depth in Chapter 8.

➤ *Short-term insomnia* lasts up to two or three weeks and often develops as a result of emotional stress. Job changes, divorce, serious illness, financial troubles, or the death of a loved one can all contribute to short-term insomnia. Short-term insomnia may resolve itself, but often re-quires some kind of psychological therapy or medical advice in order to keep it from becoming a chronic problem.

➤ *Chronic insomnia* lasts longer than a few weeks and yields poor sleep almost every night or for several nights during each month. It is debilitating, frustrating, and self-perpetuating. If a medical problem or clinical sleep disorder doesn't cause it, you may be able to trace it to an unresolved psychological upset or trauma. Stress-related insomnia—that is, insomnia exacerbated by the fear of not being able to sleep—often becomes chronic as well. So, too, does insomnia caused by poor *sleep hygiene* habits.

No matter what type of insomnia you suffer from, we'll show you some safe and effective strategies to help ease your problem. But first let's find out exactly how your insomnia presents itself.

The "When" of Insomnia

Fortunately, there are very few people—even those who define themselves as helpless insomniacs—who *never* go to sleep throughout an entire night. Generally speaking, insomniacs fall into one of three categories:

➤ *Delayed sleepers* have trouble falling asleep once they get into bed. Generally speaking, Owls tend to develop this problem more often than Larks, especially when they're trying to get to sleep earlier than usual in order to wake up earlier.

➤ *Frequent awakeners* are disturbed from sleep at least once and often several times during the night. In most cases, a sleep disorder like apnea or a medical problem like chronic pain triggers this type of insomnia. Stress may also cause someone to wake up often during the night.

➤ *Early awakeners* find themselves waking up very early in the morning—generally before 5:00 a.m.—before having had enough sleep. Larks tend to find themselves in this situation more often than their Owl counterparts, especially as they start to become tired and fall asleep earlier in the evening to make up for the loss of sleep in the morning. By switching on the lights each morning (see Chapter 11), they make the awakening even earlier the next night.

Wake Up!

If you have trouble sleeping after suffering an emotional trauma, talk to your doctor. Under this type of special circumstance, taking medication under close medical supervision may be appropriate. Otherwise, your ability to cope with the trauma may well become hampered by the effects of sleep deprivation.

Night Owl Wisdom

Sleep hygiene refers to the daily habits that surround sleep, such as establishing a regular evening routine to prepare you for sleep, eating your last big meal several hours before bedtime, and creating a quiet, comfortable sleep environment.

Unfortunately, once the natural patterns of "Owls" and "Larks" become disrupted, chronic sleep deprivation can result, especially if these natural patterns are very rigid.

Take Oliver, for instance. Oliver is naturally an extreme Owl. In the best of all possible worlds, Oliver would stay awake until 2 a.m. and sleep until 8 or 9 in the morning (he feels best on about 6 hours of sleep per night). Oliver prefers to work at tasks that take the most concentration between 10 p.m. and 1 a.m. However, he does find it relatively easy to shift his bedtime back about 2 hours, so that he falls asleep at about midnight and wakes up at 6 or 7 a.m. This would give him plenty of time to get to work by 10 a.m. or so. Since Oliver works for a company that allows its employees to make their own hours most of the time, Oliver's sleep pattern works well for him.

Oliver can easily get into trouble, however, if he is called into an early morning meeting—one that convenes at 8 or 9 a.m. If he is unable to fall asleep earlier than usual the night before, he will wake up feeling tired in the morning and drag through the day. By 8 or 9 p.m. he'll be so exhausted that he will fall asleep at that time. If he could sleep straight through to morning, it would be okay, but instead, he usually wakes up—fresh as a daisy—at midnight and then can't fall asleep again until near dawn. He'll also get into the same kind of trouble if he loses sight of the time and simply works until his natural rhythm kicks in, which could be as late as 2 or 3 a.m.

Once such a pattern is established, the only way Oliver can break it is by making sure that he naps for just an hour at around 8 p.m. and then works until his regular sleep time of midnight or so. If he then sleeps through to his regular wake-up time of 6 or 7 a.m., he'll be back on his regular schedule.

Letitia, on the other hand, is a Lark, and a rather rigid one to boot. Lights out for Letitia is usually around 10 p.m. and her wake-up time around 4 a.m. (four complete sleep cycles). Having very good *Nap-Ability*, Letitia easily adds to her sleep during the day by taking either a few 10-minute catnaps or, if she's feeling especially sleep deprived, a full hour-and-a-half nap (one full sleep cycle).

Letitia can get into trouble with her sleep patterns, however, if something keeps her up much later than normal. Being a Rigid Lark, Letitia won't naturally continue to sleep until she gets her regular 6 hours, but

Just for You!

Timing is everything: If you're not going to get your normal number of hours, time your wake-up so that you don't interrupt a 90-minute sleep cycle right in the middle. Instead of falling asleep 7 hours before you have to get up, for instance, stay up another hour. You'll get one less hour, but you'll complete four whole sleep cycles rather than interrupt the last one, waking up groggy and tired. Try it and see if it helps improve the way you feel the next day.

Night Owl Wisdom

Remember, **Nap-Ability** refers to how easily, not how regularly, you nap. Those with great Nap Ability can nap both in anticipation of a need to sleep (knowing they're going to have a late night) and to make up for a sleep loss.

will wake up promptly at 4 a.m. no matter how little she's slept. If she can't catch a nap during the workday, she'll end up being too tired and edgy to go to sleep earlier than her usual time. The fact that she usually grabs more sugar snacks and caffeinated beverages during the day to give her a little boost doesn't help either.

Once overtired and stressed, Letitia finds herself waking up earlier and earlier—sometimes as early as 3 a.m.—and cutting back more and more on her sleep until she's exhausted. Only by taking a long, restful $1^1/_2$-hour nap at least 5 hours before her normal bedtime can she break out of this cycle that would eventually lead to chronic insomnia. Interestingly, once she has taken such a nap, she finds she has reset her sleep/wake cycle and that night will stay up an extra half hour but sleep through to 5:30 or 6 a.m. (that is, she'll get five instead of four full sleep cycles).

Do you recognize yourself in either Oliver (the Owl) or Letitia (the Lark)? Could your sleep problem be linked to a disruption in your natural rhythm? Of course, the examples cited here are just two of the many types of insomnia patterns—and we'll be describing others as we go along. If you're a Regular Robin, for instance, a disruption on either end of your day can lead to difficulties.

In any case, it's important for you to evaluate your sleep patterns in this way as you consider the source of your current difficulties—and we'll remind you of that approach often. In the meantime, let's revisit the subject of sleep deprivation and what it really means to your life and your health.

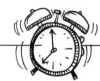

Wake Up!

It's a myth that everyone *needs* 8 hours of sleep every night. You might thrive on just 5 or 6. If those five or six happen to fall between 10 p.m. and 4 a.m. then—unless it profoundly interferes with other priorities—you might be best advised to simply go with the flow. Get out of bed at 4 a.m., tackle some work, read, or get your daily exercise out of the way.

The Symptoms of Exhaustion

Think of the last time that you had a bad night's sleep or no sleep at all. The next day, you probably felt a little weak, a little off the mark, maybe even nauseous and headachy. If you're lucky, you got to bed a bit earlier the next night and woke up feeling refreshed once again.

But if you suffer from insomnia, if it takes you even an extra hour to fall asleep or if you wake up just an hour too early, the toll on your body can be significant within a very short amount of time. Indeed, when you deprive yourself of sleep, the total amount of sleep loss accumulates over days. Fortunately, when you're really tired, your sleep becomes more efficient—that is, you spend more time in Stages 3 and 4 of deep sleep, thereby making up for lost sleep more quickly. (Remember Letitia, our Lark example: She can make up for a whole work-week's worth of lesser-than-normal amounts of sleep with just one $1/_2$-hour nap during the weekend.)

Needless to say, the symptoms listed above are both unpleasant and dangerous. We cited some statistics in Chapter 1 about the relationship between daytime tiredness and auto accidents, and sleep deprivation and illness (especially among shift workers). Sleepy people are also more likely to gain weight and suffer from lack of stamina.

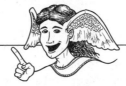

Morpheus Says

Thomas Reilly and Mark Piercy of the Center for Sport and Exercise Sciences at John Moores University in Liverpool tested weight lifters whose nightly sleep had been reduced to 3 hours. By the second night, their ability to bench press, leg press, and dead–lift weight had all deteriorated. As their sleep debts accumulated, their performances continued to suffer.

The Influence of Lifestyle: A Quiz

Barring any medical problems or special circumstances like night-shift work or time-zone travel, you should be able to get the sleep you need quite naturally. But if you're reading this book, chances are you're failing in this area.

Why? Our best guess is that something in your daily life is disrupting your physiology, preventing your body from easing its way into sleep—thus allowing the body and brain to recover and renew themselves before facing the next day's challenges.

To find out what in your day-to-day life is getting in the way of a good night's sleep, take the following quiz.

The Influence of Lifestyle Quiz

Part A: Lifestyle Habits

Answer "Yes" or "No" to the following statements.

1. I am at least 20 pounds overweight.
   Yes _____ No _____
2. I frequently eat dinner within 2 hours of bedtime.
   Yes _____ No _____
3. I drink caffeinated beverages, often after 6 p.m.
   Yes _____ No _____

4. I lead a sedentary life.
   Yes _____ No _____

5. Most of my exercise periods occur within 2 hours of bedtime.
   Yes _____ No _____

Part B: The Impact of Stress

Answer the following statements 1) Usually, 2) Sometimes, or 3) Rarely.

1. I end the day feeling unsatisfied with my accomplishments. _____

2. During the day, I don't feel I have much control over my work and personal life. _____

3. I don't practice yoga, meditation, or other relaxation strategy. _____

4. I worry about getting to sleep. _____

5. I'm unable to shut out thoughts about responsibilities, unfinished business, or other worries during the evening and night. _____

Part C: Appreciating Proper Sleep Hygiene

Answer "Yes" or "No" to the following statements.

1. I watch television or do paperwork in bed before sleep.
   Yes _____ No _____

2. My mattress is more than 5 years old and sags.
   Yes _____ No _____

3. Noise and light have easy access into my bedroom.
   Yes _____ No _____

4. I suffer from allergies and haven't taken steps to remove my allergy triggers from my bedroom.
   Yes _____ No _____

5. I rarely go to bed at the same time or follow the same routine before bed.
   Yes _____ No _____

Part D: The Pharmaceutical Industry

Answer "Yes" or "No" to the following statements.

1. I take prescription sleeping pills on many or most nights.
   Yes _____ No _____

2. I use over-the-counter sleep remedies more than once a week.
   Yes _____ No _____

3. If I don't use medication, I cannot sleep well.
   Yes _____ No _____

4. I use herbal potions and teas to help me relax.
   Yes _____ No _____

5. I take melatonin supplements on a regular basis.
   Yes _____ No _____

Part E: The Power of Light

Answer "Yes" or "No" to the following statements.

1. I rarely get outside in the sunlight during the day.
   Yes _____ No _____

2. My office has no windows that let in sunlight.
   Yes _____ No _____

3. My energy level diminishes during the fall and winter.
   Yes _____ No _____

4. If I get up and outside in the light early in the morning, I go to sleep earlier at night.
   Yes _____ No _____

5. My bedroom never gets completely dark.
   Yes _____ No _____

Part F: To Nap or Not to Nap

Answer the following statements 1) Usually, 2) Sometimes, or 3) Rarely.

1. I feel sleepy but am unable to sleep during the day. _____

2. When I nap, it is typically for longer than 30 minutes but less than $1^1/_2$ hours. _____

3. I nap after I get home from work, around 6 p.m. _____

4. I don't have the time and place to nap at work. _____

5. I wake up from a nap feeling paralyzed and groggy. _____

Sleep Solutions

How did you do on the quiz? Can you see how your daily habits or nighttime routine may be interfering with how well you sleep and how much sleep you get? Let's explore the possibilities. Check back over your answers to the appropriate part of the quiz as you read the following sections.

Part A: Lifestyle Habits

If you answered yes to even one of these questions, you may be able to trace your sleep problem to your diet or exercise habits. Indeed, knowing when to eat, what to eat, and what substances to avoid—namely caffeine and alcohol—in order to optimize your sleep is an important place for any insomniac to start. Exercise habits, including when and how much you exercise, also have an impact on your ability to sleep, and sleep well. You'll find more information about this aspect of sleep hygiene in Chapter 7.

Part B: The Impact of Stress

If you often answered with usually, you need to find a way to reduce the amount of stress and tension you feel on a day-to-day basis. As you'll discover when you read Chapter 8, your body produces certain chemicals in response to stress, and these body chemicals can interfere with proper sleep patterns. Learning to reduce stress levels is not as hard as you might think, as we'll show you later on.

Part C: Appreciating Proper Sleep Hygiene

You've probably already guessed that if you answered yes to one or more questions in this part, your bedroom may have become your worst enemy when it comes to sleep. In Chapter 9, we'll show you how to create a sleep-enhancing bedroom—starting with the bed and working around the room.

Part D: The Pharmaceutical Industry

If you've answered yes to even one of these questions, you must pay special attention to Chapter 10. Prescription and over-the-counter sleep remedies have a definite and useful purpose when it comes to solving sleep problems, but they must be used with great care and often under a doctor's watchful eye. Herbs and hormone supplements like melatonin can also be helpful, but they, too, have their risks and side effects.

Part E: The Power of Light

Did you answer even one question with a yes? If you're like most modern Americans, you're tied to your desk or in the house with the kids from dawn till dusk. Since the natural rise and fall of the sun is our primary Zeitgeber ("timegiver"), it's no wonder we have such difficulty attaining regular, good sleep. In Chapter 11, we'll show you how light can become your best friend in your quest for a good night's sleep.

Part F: To Nap or Not to Nap

How many questions provoked a "Usually" response from you? The more 1's you wrote down, the more likely it is that you've never made napping a successful part of your sleep pattern—which would be just fine if you were also sleeping well during the night. Since you're having trouble, we'll show you in Chapter 13 how a daytime nap can help you get the sleep you need.

In the next several chapters, we outline some healthy habits that will help you get a better night's sleep. If you have a particular problem—say with exercise or stress reduction—feel free to skip to the chapter that you feel most applies to you. We suggest, though, that you read straight through. You're sure to find useful and interesting information in every chapter. We start with creating an eating and exercise plan designed to optimize your sleep.

The Least You Need to Know

➤ Sleep problems have many causes and many different solutions.

➤ It's important to be aware of your sleep type and its impact on your vulnerability to certain kinds of insomnia.

➤ Examining your daily habits is a good place to look for sleep-related solutions.

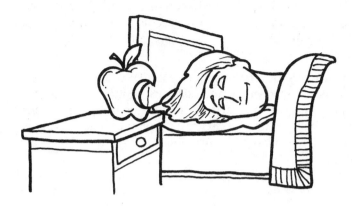

Chapter 7

Healthy Habits

In This Chapter

➤ Understanding the effect of daily habits on sleep

➤ Exploring the substances in food that promote sleep

➤ Balancing the risks and benefits of caffeine and alcohol

➤ Learning about the sleep-inducing power of exercise

Bad habits: You probably have one or two that you struggle with (we all do), and chances are they involve one of two areas (and sometimes both) of our lives: diet and exercise. Some of us eat too much of the wrong kind of food or too little of the right kind. Others of us get too little exercise, or we exercise at the wrong time. And then there are those of us with both bad habits—and you know who you are!

Unfortunately, in addition to messing with your waistline and threatening your health in myriad ways, a failure to establish healthy eating and exercise patterns can also affect your ability to sleep well. The good news is that by making certain regular changes in these areas of your daily life, you significantly increase your chances of sleeping well. In this chapter, we'll show you how.

You Sleep What You Eat

Although it's probably not the first thing you think of when identifying risk factors for insomnia, your diet does indeed influence the way you sleep. First, healthy people generally enjoy healthy sleep—or at least they stand a much better chance of doing so than those who are less healthy. Second, the choices you make about how much and what kinds of food you eat in the hours before bedtime have a direct impact on how well you're able to sleep that night. After all, when you think about it, food is made up of chemicals that can act on the body just the way a drug might work. But we'll get to that part of the equation a little later in this chapter.

For now, if you're like most Americans, your relationship to your daily diet is perhaps not the healthiest. Nearly half of us are overweight, and our consumption of high-fat, calorie-laden, nutrient-poor foods continues unabated. Although a definite correlation cannot be drawn as yet, it's hard to believe that the rise in sleep problems of all types is completely unrelated to this fall in dietary standards! We'll help you figure out if there's room for improvement in your daily diet.

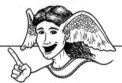

Morpheus Says

A 1994 article in the *Journal of the American Medical Association* pointed out that more than 33 percent of American men and women were currently obese, or weighed 20 percent or more over their optimal body weight. Furthermore, a 1995 study reported in the *New York Times* found that the number of overweight children in the United States had more than doubled over the last 30 years.

Eating for Health

Needless to say, there are literally hundreds of books that outline healthy eating plans and discuss nutrition in depth and with authority, so we won't even attempt to do that here. But since diet is an integral part of a healthy lifestyle, and being healthy encourages better sleep, we'll offer a few tips that might help you develop a sensible approach to your daily diet:

➤ *Maintain a healthy weight.* Heart disease, high blood pressure, stroke, diabetes, cancer—at all ages and stages of life, being overweight contributes to these and other health problems. Being overweight can also interfere with your ability to get a good night's sleep. For one thing, it puts you at higher risk for Obstructive Sleep Apnea, a sleep disorder we discuss in Chapter 14. Depending on how much extra girth you've got, you may also find it more difficult to find a comfortable sleeping position. It's also more likely that you don't get enough exercise, since weight gain and a sedentary life often go hand in hand.

➤ *Choose healthy foods.* Choose fresh fruits and vegetables, whole-grain breads and pasta, and low-fat proteins (fish, chicken, beans, and tofu) when planning your meals. Avoid fatty, processed, and preservative-rich foods as much as possible. In addition to causing many other problems, they also increase the chances you'll develop heartburn, ulcers, and other gastrointestinal disturbances that contribute to sleep disturbances.

➤ *Balance your diet.* The biggest diet mistake made by Americans is obsessing on, and indulging in, fat-free foods, which leads us to load up on carbohydrates. Unbalanced meals high in carbohydrates stimulate insulin production and signal to the body to synthesize and store fat. Including limited fats, balanced with protein and some carbohydrates in moderation, is the most effective way to control your weight.

➤ *Structure your mealtimes.* Eating on the run and skipping or forgetting to eat meals are endemic bad habits in our all-too-busy society. But eating your meals on a regular schedule will help keep all of your internal circadian rhythms up and running, including your sleep/wake patterns.

➤ *Make dinner your lightest meal.* Eating a heavy or large meal within a few hours before bedtime sets your body up for a rough night of sleep. Try eating a small amount—about three to four ounces—of protein such as chicken, along with a serving of complex carbohydrates such as whole-wheat pasta or a baked sweet potato. Avoid eating high-sugar foods before bedtime; they'll only make it harder for you to fall asleep. However, don't go to bed hungry, either, which could be a recipe for disaster as well.

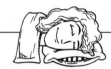

Sleep on it

Developing a relatively set schedule for your mealtimes, exercise sessions, and other routine day-to-day activities will help you in your quest for regular, restful sleep. Your body runs on an internal clock, and the more you make use of external Zeitgebers (timegivers), the more likely you'll be to maintain a healthy sleep/wake pattern.

The Sleep Promoters

Hungry for a late-night snack? Well, if you have trouble sleeping, you may be able to help alleviate the problem by making more careful choices when you're choosing your munchies.

Optimally, you want to choose foods that contain the amino acid tryptophan. Tryptophan is important for sleep because it is the precursor of the neurotransmitter called *serotonin*, one of the body's "sleep" chemicals (and a primary neurotransmitter involved in regulating your moods). One of the functions of serotonin is to slow down nerve activity, therefore inducing sleep. Tryptophan is also the precursor of melatonin, the "sleep hormone" that helps set the stage for sleep.

A glass of warm milk contains tryptophan—that's why it's often prescribed as a sleep aid (unless you're lactose-intolerant and the resulting upset stomach would keep you awake). Other foods high in tryptophan include peanut butter, dates, figs, rice, tuna, turkey (which is one of the reasons you get sleepy after Thanksgiving dinner!), and yogurt. It takes about an hour for tryptophan to reach the brain after you consume it, so plan your snack wisely. It's also possible to take tryptophan in the form of a supplement, a fact we'll discuss at more length in Chapter 10.

In addition to timing the consumption of tryptophan-rich foods, you may also want to look at whether you're receiving enough vitamins and minerals in your regular diet. Certain vitamins and minerals affect your ability to sleep and the quality of the sleep you get. Among the most often cited nutrients related to sleep are the following:

Night Owl Wisdom

Serotonin is a neurotransmitter (a chemical messenger) important in a wide variety of brain functions, including the regulation of moods. People who suffer from depression, as well as depression-related insomnia, often have deficient levels of serotonin in the brain.

Wake Up!

Although consuming tryptophan in the foods you eat poses no health risk whatsoever—and may help you set your body's stage for sleep—tryptophan supplements can be dangerous. Please discuss the matter with your physician, and be sure to read the section about tryptophan supplements in Chapter 10.

➤ *Vitamin B complex.* In addition to working directly to promote a healthy nervous system (one that can relax as well as it can stimulate), the B vitamins regulate the body's use of tryptophan and other amino acids. They appear to be especially helpful for people with depression who also have trouble sleeping. Among the B vitamins that strongly influence sleep are B3 (niacin), B5 (panthothenic acid), B6 (pyridoxine), B12 (cyancobalamin), folic acid, and inositol. Be aware, however, that some people experience a paradoxical effect when it comes to the B vitamins and sleep—for them, taking supplements has a stimulatory rather than relaxing effect on the nervous system.

➤ *Calcium and magnesium.* Working together, as they should, these two minerals not only help to keep bones and teeth strong, but also act as natural relaxants. Calcium, in particular, helps the body release tryptophan, which helps the body manufacture melatonin. And, as a 1978 study at the University of Alabama showed, even a minor calcium deficiency can lead to insomnia due to muscle tension.

➤ *Copper and iron.* A deficiency in iron or copper can cause poor sleep, primarily because of their effects on the production of certain neurotransmitters. Copper, for instance, is necessary for the production of norepinephrine, and iron helps produce dopamine. It is especially important for you to get your doctor's advice before taking supplements of either copper or iron, as too much of these minerals can cause serious side effects.

➤ *Zinc.* Some research indicates that a mild zinc deficiency causes some infants to wake up fussy frequently during the night, and it may be that some adults can benefit from taking more zinc as well. You can take zinc supplements without hesitation for a few weeks to see if your sleep improves, but DO NOT give your infant or toddler zinc without first checking with his or her pediatrician.

As you can see, the substances you put, or fail to put, into your body may influence your ability to sleep. However, if you decide to take supplements or change your diet, you might want to add a category to your Sleep Log (discussed in Chapter 5) that tracks the changes you make and the effect they have. Make one change at a time, then write down its effect, if any, on your sleep over the next few weeks.

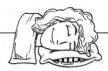

Sleep on it

Before you start taking more than the minimum daily requirement of any vitamin or mineral, check with your doctor. Too much of a good thing can be harmful to your general health and your sleep. Your doctor can help you determine the proper dosage of vitamin and mineral supplements. If you decide to supplement your intake, you should monitor their effect on your sleep with care.

Perhaps the biggest concern when it comes to diet and sleep has nothing to do with the food you eat, but rather with the beverages you drink. Indeed, two common substances found in popular drinks—caffeine and alcohol—are major, but avoidable, sleep bandits. (As we'll discuss later, caffeine is found not only in coffee, tea, and cola but also in many foods.)

The Caffeine Connection

In the United States alone, more than 80 percent of adults consume caffeine on regular basis and, on average, ingest the caffeine equivalent of about three cups of coffee a day (about 280 milligrams). A select few of us (about 20 percent) have really got it bad, consuming up to 500 mg or more.

As ubiquitous as caffeine is, it's a drug that produces intense effects on the human mind and body. For most people, the effects are pleasurable. But for others, just a little bit of caffeine on a regular basis can lead to fragmented concentration, headaches, heartburn, irritability, shakiness, chronic gastrointestinal problems, and—yes indeed—insomnia.

As you may already know, caffeine is a *stimulant*, a member of a group of alkaloids called xanthine derivatives. Other xanthine derivatives include theophylline and theobromine. All three substances act to speed up your central nervous

Night Owl Wisdom

A **stimulant** is a substance that speeds up the body's activities. Caffeine belongs to a family of stimulants found in plants called xanthine derivatives.

system. Coffee contains only caffeine, but other products may contain small amounts of theophylline and theobromine as well such as certain cold medications and colas.

What Happens...Fast!

Within 15 minutes of consuming caffeine, the drug begins to take effect. It acts to increase the amount of the hormone epinephrine (also known as adrenaline) and triggers the following biological events:

➤ An increase of heart rate and blood pressure

➤ An increase in respiration rate (because caffeine also relaxes smooth muscle tissues such as those that line the bronchial tubes)

➤ An increase in the production of stomach acid

➤ An increase in urinary output

➤ Stimulation of brain activity

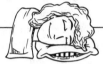

Sleep on it

If you have trouble sleeping, avoid consuming any caffeine for at least 4 hours before bedtime—even longer if you're very sensitive to its effects. If you still have insomnia, try avoiding caffeine after dinner or lunch to see if it's really the caffeine that's keeping you awake. If you're highly sensitive, you may have to cut all caffeine from your diet in order to sleep well.

The effect caffeine produces varies considerably from person to person—and that's where it gets tricky. People who are very sensitive to caffeine may find that *any* amount of the substance consumed at *any* point during the day can disrupt sleep. Others find that if they restrict their intake to the early part of the day, and certainly before dinner, they're okay. Virtually all caffeine is eliminated from the body 12 to 24 hours after it was last consumed, taking with it all its effects and side effects.

Discovering the Hidden Sources

Where does this high-octane elixir come from? Caffeine is a naturally occurring substance found in the leaves, seeds, or fruits of more than 60 different plants. The most famous caffeinated plants are coffee and cocoa beans, kola nuts, and tea leaves.

While the use of caffeine certainly has a place in the treatment of a sleep problem's main side effect—daytime drowsiness, which we'll discuss in more depth in Chapter 12—it is one of the very last things you want coursing through your body when you're trying to fall asleep.

What you may not realize is how much caffeine most of us really consume on a daily basis. Take the following quiz to see how much of this often-hidden ingredient you consume in your diet.

Caffeine Test

Substance	Milligrams (mg) of Caffeine		Number of Servings		Total Mg
Coffee/Tea					
Per 5 oz. Serving					
Drip coffee	130	×	_____	=	_____
Percolated coffee	110	×	_____	=	_____
Instant coffee	60	×	_____	=	_____
Decaf coffee	2	×	_____	=	_____
Tea (weak brew)	40	×	_____	=	_____
Tea (medium brew)	60	×	_____	=	_____
Tea (strong brew)	80	×	_____	=	_____
Soft Drinks—Regular					
Per 12 oz. Serving					
Coca-Cola	65	×	_____	=	_____
Pepsi-Cola	43	×	_____	=	_____
Dr Pepper	61	×	_____	=	_____
Mountain Dew	52	×	_____	=	_____
Shasta Cola	42	×	_____	=	_____
RC Cola	50	×	_____	=	_____
Jolt Cola	71	×	_____	=	_____
Soft Drinks—Diet					
Per 12 oz. Serving					
Diet Coke	45	×	_____	=	_____
Tab	44	×	_____	=	_____
Diet Pepsi	34	×	_____	=	_____
Pepsi Light	34	×	_____	=	_____
Diet Dr Pepper	37	×	_____	=	_____
Diet-Rite cola	34	×	_____	=	_____

continues

Continued

Substance	Milligrams (mg) of Caffeine		Number of Servings		Total Mg
Over the Counter Medicines					
Per tablet or capsule					
Excedrin	65	×	_____	=	_____
Anacin	32	×	_____	=	_____
Aspirin (plain)	0	×	_____	=	_____
Vanquish	33	×	_____	=	_____
Bromo-Seltzer	32	×	_____	=	_____
Cope tablets	32	×	_____	=	_____
Empirin	32	×	_____	=	_____
Midol	32	×	_____	=	_____
Over-the-Counter Medicines—Cold/Allergy					
Dristan	16	×	_____	=	_____
Sinarest	30	×	_____	=	_____
Corybian-D	30	×	_____	=	_____
Stimulants					
No-Doz	100	×	_____	=	_____
Vivarin	200	×	_____	=	_____
Chocolate (per 1 ounce, except where noted)					
Baking	35	×	_____	=	_____
Dark	20	×	_____	=	_____
Chocolate cake	14	×	_____	=	_____
Milk chocolate (2 ounces)	12	×	_____	=	_____
Cocoa beverage (6 ounces)	10	×	_____	=	_____
Pudding pop (2 ounces)	4	×	_____	=	_____
Brownie (with nuts)	6	×	_____	=	_____
			Daily Total		_____

Add each amount to come up with a daily total. How do you rate? Remember that reaction to caffeine varies from one individual to the next. These ranges serve as a general guideline:

Total Milligrams Per Day	Status
0–250	No problem for most people
250–500	High; reduce intake
Over 500	Very high; take immediate action

Copyright © 1998 by Circadian Information Limited Partnership. Reproduced with permission. All rights reserved.

Cutting Back

If you're a big coffee or caffeinated-soda drinker, the biggest obstacles you face are the withdrawal symptoms that often occur when you cut back your daily consumption of caffeine from the amount your body has come to expect. When your body doesn't get what it needs to start its engine, the following caffeine withdrawal symptoms may occur:

➤ Headache

➤ Drowsiness

➤ Fatigue

➤ Irritability

➤ Depression

➤ Nausea

➤ Flu-like symptoms, such as muscle aches and fever

The best way to avoid experiencing these symptoms is to slowly cut back on your caffeine consumption, using less and less every day. The following tips will help you get started:

➤ *Keep track.* Once you figure out how much caffeine you consume and decide to cut back, keep track of the effects of reduced consumption in your daily Sleep Log.

➤ *Check labels.* As the earlier quiz may have revealed, you could be consuming far more caffeine than you realize. Make sure you know how much caffeine is in the foods you eat, the beverages you drink, and the medication you take.

➤ *Take your time.* If you'd like to reduce the amount of caffeine you drink—or eliminate it from your diet altogether—it's best to do so slowly and spread it out over time by reducing the amount you consume by 20 percent each week. (For example, if you drink five cups of coffee a day, cut back by just one cup a day the first week, then another cup the next week, and so on until you start to feel better.)

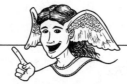

Morpheus Says

A study of adolescents with insomnia, reported in the journal *Pediatrics*, shows that you're never too young to have a caffeine-related sleep problem. If you have a child who's having trouble sleeping, check the amount of caffeine he or she is consuming in soft drinks and chocolate products. It may be time to cut back.

➤ *Switch to decaf (or low-caf) beverages gradually.* If you're a coffee drinker, you can progressively switch from regular to decaf by mixing them before brewing. Mix in a higher proportion of decaf every day. Or switch to tea, which has less caffeine than coffee.

➤ *Find healthy substitutes.* Try Postum or Pero, grain-based instant beverages that provide the richness and warmth of coffee, but without the caffeine. It may take a while to get used to the difference, but when you adapt, you'll be pleased.

➤ *Water, water everywhere.* Water is one of the most underrated health foods in the world—the non-caffeinated kind, anyway—and we urge you to drink as much of it as you can. Water helps flush out body toxins and hydrates your skin and other tissues.

➤ *Take a break.* To cope with the dips in energy you may feel as you taper off your caffeine consumption, try taking a brisk walk outside or performing some easy stretches to get your blood flowing. Deep breathing exercises send oxygen to the blood and brain. If you're really sleepy and can manage it, take a nap—another highly underrated, healthful activity. We'll give you more tips for staying awake and feeling refreshed, even if you haven't solved your sleep problem yet, in Chapter 12. In the meantime, there's another substance linked to problems with sleep that many people consume on a regular basis: alcohol.

The Alcohol Trap

A brandy before bedtime is one of the oldest prescriptions for a good night's sleep. Unfortunately, for most people, drinking alcohol anywhere close to bedtime may act to disturb rather than aid sleep.

While alcohol may help you fall asleep faster, it can significantly diminish the quality of sleep you obtain during the night. For example, having alcohol in your system can cause you to wake up prematurely—sometimes with an urgent need to urinate. It can also reduce the time you spend in REM sleep (see Chapter 3). Drinking too much alcohol is also associated with an increase in snoring and sleep apnea.

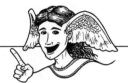

Morpheus Says

Alcohol increases the severity of sleep apnea and snoring primarily by relaxing the muscles in the throat, as well as by suppressing the body's "awakening" systems. A study of 20 men between the ages of 20 and the mid-60s found that those who were given four shots of vodka within an hour of bedtime had five times more frequent episodes of sleep apnea than men who consumed no alcohol.

However, as is true for caffeine, the effects of alcohol vary considerably among individuals. Many people enjoy a glass of wine or two with dinner and suffer no ill effects. Some even manage quite well having a liqueur or brandy within an hour or two before bedtime. Others, however, are unable to tolerate any alcohol in their systems and, therefore, should avoid it for several hours before they try to sleep.

A second consideration comes into play when it comes to alcohol, and that is dependence. There's quite a difference between enjoying a nightcap before bed and *needing* a nightcap in order to sleep. Once you start to cross over that line, you may need some help in cutting back on the amount of alcohol you drink on a daily basis, or eliminating alcohol altogether.

Wake Up!

Avoid alcohol when you're sleep-deprived. Sleep deprivation greatly magnifies the effects of alcohol, and just one drink could make you feel drunk and prevent you from taking proper care while driving or performing other routine tasks.

If you have any questions about how alcohol may be affecting your sleep—or any aspect of your life, for that matter—talk to your doctor about it. In the meantime, it's a good idea for you to carefully track how much you drink and how you sleep on the nights you drink. If, after a few weeks, you see that you've established an unhealthy pattern, it's time to take control.

Indeed, there are many other, healthier ways to wind down than drinking alcohol. One of the best methods is exercise—a sure-fire stress reliever and sleep aid.

Work It Out

The benefits of regular exercise are almost too many to mention. In addition to reducing your risk of developing heart disease, high blood pressure, some kinds of cancer, and many other diseases, exercise helps improve your mood and reduce stress. As a wonderful side effect, it also improves the quality of your sleep.

The Sleep-Promoting Benefits of Exercise

Contrary to popular belief, exercise doesn't help you sleep by making your body tired. People who have trouble sleeping aren't helped even when they are physically exhausted. Instead, exercise alleviates physical stress and certain medical disorders that may affect sleep. Here are just a few of the reasons you might want to add exercise to your life if you're having trouble getting a good night's sleep:

➤ *Exercise helps you fall asleep faster.* In one recent study, a regular exercise routine cut the time it took to fall asleep in half—from 28 to 14 minutes. The study focused on a group of formerly sedentary people who had completed a 16-week program of moderate exercise.

➤ Exercise helps you sleep longer. The same study found that exercise added an average of more than 45 minutes to the participants' main sleep blocks.

➤ *Exercise improves sleep quality.* To wake up feeling refreshed, you need to spend a good proportion of your time in bed in deep sleep. A 1994 study found that people who completed an aerobic training course experienced a 33 percent increase in sleep Stages 3 and 4—the slow-wave sleep that is the deepest type of sleep.

➤ *Exercise can help shift your biological clock.* Recent research suggests that exercise offers a bonus for people who must be up at night, either for work or for personal obligations. It shifts circadian rhythms, indirectly leading to a better mood and alertness on the work schedule or shift you choose to follow. In Chapters 14 and 15, on night work and time-zone travel, we'll discuss this subject in more depth.

Just for You!

If you're an extreme Owl, getting your exercise outside in the sunlight early in the day can help shift your biological clock forward, so that you'll get up a little earlier in the day and go to bed a little earlier at night—and feel better doing it!

Making Exercise a Part of Your Life

There's no question about it: It's just as hard to incorporate a new positive habit into your life as it is to break a old bad one. And if you're sedentary, making exercise a regular part of your life will take a little work, a lot of commitment, and some perseverance. The benefits, on the other hand, will be well worth the effort.

When it comes to exercising in order to increase your chances of getting a good night's sleep, it's best to focus on increasing the amount of cardiovascular exercise you get. That means walking, running, playing singles tennis, swimming, and bicycling, to name just a few activities. At the same time, if you prefer yoga and weight-training, by all means, start there. Whatever you do to increase your physical fitness and help yourself relieve stress will improve the quality and quantity of sleep you obtain.

Here are a few tips to get you started:

➤ *Start slowly.* Don't overdo. If you try to put in 2 hours a day every day during your first week exercising, you'll only end up sore and discouraged—and *very* unlikely to want to work out the next week. The best way to stick to exercising is to start small and build gradually: 20 to 30 minutes are all you need to start improving your level of fitness.

➤ *Time exercise sessions with care.* If getting to sleep at night is difficult for you, try exercising in the late afternoon or early evening. Exercise helps to raise the body temperature, helping set the stage for sleep. DO NOT exercise within 3 hours of bedtime, however. You'll only stimulate your muscles and increase your alertness, making it more difficult than ever for you to fall asleep. If stress reduction is your motivation, then exercise whenever you can fit in an activity on a regular basis. Some people find exercising in the late afternoon is best, since muscular performance is best and tolerance for physical stress appears to be highest at this time.

➤ *Set realistic goals.* If you've been sedentary for a number of months or years, deciding to train for next month's marathon by running 10 miles every morning would be counterproductive and even dangerous to your health. After failing to meet this unrealistic goal, or straining your muscles trying to do so, you'd become frustrated and probably decide not to exercise at all. Instead, set goals you know you can meet or perhaps ones just barely within your reach. Achieving them will give you a sense of pride and self-confidence that's sure to keep you motivated.

➤ *Add variety.* To alleviate boredom, try alternating activities. Take a dance class one session, bicycle outside the next, or perform yoga postures every other morning. By varying your routine, you're more likely to keep it going.

➤ *Seek convenience.* Another hint to help you stick to an exercise program is to eliminate as many excuses as possible for not exercising. If you join a health club that is open only during hours you're at work, for instance, then obviously you're setting yourself up to fail. Scheduling times to exercise—and treating your exercise times as if they were business appointments—is often the only way to incorporate aerobic activity into your lifestyle.

➤ *Find a support group.* For most of us, there comes a time when motivation sags and we lose interest in exercise. When this happens—preferably *before* this happens—enlist a friend or loved one to join you in your quest for fitness.

Timing Is Everything

It's never too late to make positive changes in your life. If you're having trouble falling or staying asleep, now is the time to look at the components of your daily diet or exercise habits that might be keeping you up at night. We hope this chapter has helped explain some of the risks and benefits involved with certain food substances, as well as how exercise influences your ability to sleep.

Next, we'll show you another aspect of your life that has a direct impact on sleep: Stress.

The Least You Need to Know

➤ Your daily eating and exercise habits influence the quality of your sleep.

➤ It's important to understand the negative effect that caffeine and alcohol can have on sleep and then to monitor your intake of these substances to see how they affect you.

➤ You can help yourself get a better night's sleep by exercising on a regular basis.

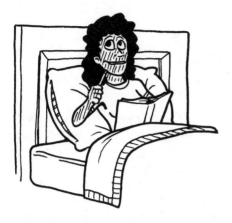

Chapter 8

Stress Reduction 101

Stress, tension, worry: This triumvirate of emotions may well be one of the reasons so many Americans find it hard to get a good night's sleep these days. As you'll discover in this chapter, the very last thing your body wants to do—biologically speaking—is to shut down and fall asleep when you feel stressed and upset. In fact, the stress response actually creates a chemical barrier to sleep by producing hormones that act to keep you alert and ready for action.

Although your sleep problem may be unrelated to excess stress—and that's something you may have to determine through trial and error—it certainly won't hurt you to think about how you cope with your day-to-day challenges. Stress not only has strong connections to sleep disruption, but is also linked to a host of other health problems, including heart disease, hypertension, allergies, depression, and anxiety—in short, many of the same chronic illnesses that themselves contribute to sleep problems.

In this chapter, we'll help you gain a better understanding of what goes on in your body when you feel stress, tension, and worry. We'll help you discover what triggers your own stress response and give you some tips for alleviating those feelings. Once you've dealt with your own stress you may find your sleep problem has disappeared, or at least become more manageable.

The Stress-Insomnia Cycle

You should know, right from the start, that many people with insomnia—and you could be one of them—get themselves into a vicious circle when it comes to stress. After experiencing a few nights of unsettled sleep for any reason, stress-related or not, you suddenly become most worried about not being able to sleep.

You toss and turn, afraid that the one thing you want to do most—close your eyes and fall asleep—is the very thing you won't be able to do—not this night, not any night. You start to think about how you'll feel the next morning, when you have to face another day feeling groggy, cranky, and out-of-sorts. You imagine that some dreadful disease is really at the heart of your sleep problem and that every night you can't sleep means it's taken a greater hold. You stare at the clock, watching the second hand sweep by, or the digits on the clock flip over, over and over again. You sit up, lie back down, fluff the pillow, and stare at the clock again. You start to sweat, your heart rate goes up—the whole idea of sleep become too difficult, too...well, too stressful.

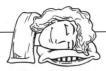

Sleep on it

If you find yourself having to leave the bedroom at night because of insomnia, choose a comfortable spot (a favorite chair or couch) to set yourself and choose a relaxing activity (like reading or knitting) rather than something stimulating (like doing your bills!). Performing a sleep-promoting ritual is as impor- tant in the middle of the night as it is before bedtime. It is crucial, however, that you go back to bed when you start to feel very sleepy, and not before.

Sound familiar? For many people with insomnia, the fear of not sleeping becomes the very trigger for the continuation of their problem. And it only gets worse when the simple sight of their bed conjures up their anxiety and tension—an all too common development. In fact, it's important to emphasize that, if you find yourself in this unhealthy cycle of stress-insomnia-more stress, you do your very best to take the struggle outside of the bedroom. Once you start relating the bedroom and your bed to frustration and fear, it becomes even more difficult to solve your sleep problem.

Instead, if you find yourself tossing and turning in frustration, get up and leave the bedroom. Read a book, knit, pet the cat—perform any activity that distracts you from the urgency of your sleep need or the worries that keep you awake. Just keep the lights turned down low to avoid resetting your biological clock and compounding the problem the next night. Only when you feel relaxed and very, very sleepy should you return to your bed. (We discuss this issue at length in Chapter 9.)

As you can see, the mind exerts a very powerful influ- ence on the entire body, and stress isn't something you can easily evaluate or moderate.

Healthy Mind/Healthy Body

We said it before back in Chapter 2: It's not possible to separate the mind from the body. Emotions and thoughts are not only biological events themselves, but they also trigger biological processes that have wide-ranging effects. That's especially true when it comes to the reaction we commonly refer to as "stress."

Although we use the word stress often, it isn't always easy to define stress or how it makes you feel. One reason is because, except in extreme situations like the death of a loved one or the threat of imminent physical harm, a clear definition of stress is not available. Everything that occurs in your life or exists in your environment is technically a stressor because it causes some internal change.

If it is very hot out, for example, your body will adjust to the increased ambient temperature by increasing heat loss through the skin by redirecting blood flow toward the skin surface and by cooling the skin with perspiration. In this instance, heat is a stressor because it poses a challenge that spurs the body to action. If you receive an unexpected and exciting assignment from your boss, the excitement the opportunity stimulates may make your heart beat faster, your muscles tense up, your palms sweat— and keep you up at night. Despite its positive impact then, the news of your assignment is a stressor because it forces a physiological reaction—one that will be described in more depth later in this chapter—to occur.

A second problem in relating stress to how we feel involves how variable our reactions to stress tend to be. Some people become outwardly aggravated over the slightest mishap, while others never blink an eye even when disaster occurs. It should be noted, however, that the outwardly calm person actually may be seething inside, perhaps with even more negative effects on his or her physiology than would be suffered by the person who expresses anger and frustration in a more open way. Indeed, it isn't the amount of stress in your life but how you react to that stress that causes the resultant illness and other negative effects.

Third, and even more significant, keep in mind that stressors vary in their effect from person to person. For some, a day spent lying on a beach is completely relaxing; for others such forced recreation is sheer torture. Again, it's how you as an individual *perceive* a situation that determines how your body reacts to it.

Wake Up!

Don't take signs that your body and mind are overloaded with stress lightly. Among the signs of stress are chronic muscle aches, gastrointestinal distress, and—yes!—insomnia. See your doctor: Stress is implicated in a host of chronic and/or life-threatening diseases, including heart disease, high blood pressure, stroke, and arthritis.

Despite the difficulties in defining and measuring stress, there is no doubt that a strong connection exists between the mind, the emotions, and all aspects of health, including how well we sleep. Before we continue the discussion about the impact of stress on sleep, let's see just what happens to the body when faced with a stressful situation.

The Physiology of Stress

If you've ever doubted that there is a connection between your emotions and your internal physiology, just think about the first time you fell in love. When you looked across the room at the object of your desire, didn't your heart beat faster? Didn't your palms sweat? Didn't you feel as if you might faint because the blood had rushed from your head to your feet as you tried to make your way to the one you loved?

In addition to infatuation, what you were feeling was fear and anticipation—of rejection, of commitment, of the unknown, perhaps even of success—and your body responded to your emotions. In a completely instinctive and interdependent way, your brain, your hormones, and your nervous system worked to prepare you to face what you perceived as a threat to your emotional, if not physical, safety.

Whether you're conscious of it or not, your body has a remarkable gift for self-preservation. When its internal balance is threatened in any way it mobilizes immediately, preparing you either to battle the impending danger or to flee from it.

We call this the "fight-or-flight response," and we're probably more used to thinking about it as occurring during times of physical danger. Let's say that seemingly out of nowhere, a bus bears down on you while you're crossing the street. Your heart starts to pound and the muscles in your legs and arms tense up. Before you know it, you're across the street, running faster and harder than you'd ever thought possible.

The sight of your loved one and the sight of the bus set off a similar chain of reactions in your body. As soon as your body perceives a threat to its sense of normalcy, it goes into action. And it does so by way of two interrelated body systems: the nervous system and the *endocrine system.*

Night Owl Wisdom

The **endocrine system** is the system in the body that produces and releases hormones, chemical messengers responsible for triggering a wide range of physiological functions.

The Hormonal Connection

Two interrelated systems, the autonomic nervous system and the endocrine system, become more active during times of stress. These two systems are so directly related to what is occurring to us emotionally and intellectually that they can be considered the physical representatives of emotions within the body.

The autonomic nervous system controls bodily functions like the heartbeat, intestinal movements, salivation, and other activities of the internal organs. One part, the sympathetic nervous system, speeds up heart rate, narrows blood vessels, and raises blood pressure during times of physical or emotional stress, while the parasympathetic nervous system works to slow down these processes when the body perceives that the stress has passed.

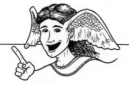

Morpheus Says

In Chinese medicine, the two parts of the autonomic nervous system represent a perfect example of the balance known as yin and yang. The sympathetic nervous system is the yang—the active, fluid aspect of life and health—while the parasympathetic is the yin—the calming, static aspect. Having the ability to bring your body back into Yin-Yang harmony after a stressful period is as important to your health as reacting immediately to perceived threats.

Directly related to nervous system activity are hormones that are secreted by the glands of the endocrine system. The glands release stress hormones into the bloodstream that in turn produce various reactions in the organs and tissues of the body. These hormones (such as epinephrine) raise the blood pressure, increase the heart rate and metabolic rate, and quicken respiration to provide more oxygen to your muscles. Other hormones, such as *cortisol*, allow the body to continue "fighting" long after the effects of the fight-or-flight response are over.

But guess what? The hormones we've just mentioned—epinephrine and cortisol—start to surge into the bloodstream as the dawn arrives. They get us ready for action in the day ahead. We're alert, we're juiced. And during the daytime our sleep hormones, particularly melatonin, are in relatively short supply. In short, we're AWAKE!

Night Owl Wisdom

Cortisol is a corticosteroid, a hormone important for normal carbohydrate metabolism as well as for the normal response to stress.

Needless to say, then, it's best to relieve as much stress as possible throughout the day and certainly before you hit the hay. Indeed, carrying the burden of stress can disrupt your life in more ways than you may know.

It's More Than Lack of Sleep

The more stress you feel, the more likely you are to engage in other behaviors detrimental to both your general health and your ability to get a good night's sleep, namely drinking alcohol, smoking cigarettes, overeating, and failing to exercise. Although you may feel that these habits help relax you, you learned in Chapter 7 that they in fact do just the opposite.

Later in this chapter, you'll learn new strategies for relieving stress in your life that emphasize bringing healthy, positive energy into your life and your body through meditation and relaxation. Combined with the exercise techniques offered in Chapter 7, these methods will work to reduce stress as well as help you break any related bad habits you've developed.

What's Keeping You Up at Night: Keeping a Daily Stress Log

Learning what aspects of your life are keeping you up at night is the first step in the process of gaining control over your health and your sleep problem. You may think you're a calm, cool, and collected individual simply because you don't explode at the drop of a hat. Or you might think that because you release your frustration by snapping at your spouse or accidentally-on-purpose deleting files from your unpleasant coworker's computer you're free and clear of stress-related problems.

And who knows? You might be right. There's no doubt that "stress" has become an all-too-common and nebulous excuse for bad behavior and bad habits. Of course, if you relieve stress as we've just described, you may end up putting your marriage in jeopardy and losing your job—stress inducers if there ever were any!

You've just read about the powerful impact stress has on the body and how that can influence your general health and your sleep patterns. Now we suggest that you take the time to track your reactions to everyday stressful occurrences. How do you feel when your train is late? Or when a bill you thought had been paid turns up overdue? We've devised a daily Stress Log that might help you identify the source of your stress and track not only your immediate reaction to the situation but also the end result. We're betting that at the end of the week, you'll discover that one way you can reduce stress is by first recognizing, and then letting go of, things you can't control—things that usually do not disrupt your life in any significant or long-lasting ways.

The following example shows how a young advertising director named Madeline first recognized, and then evaluated, the sources of her stress.

Madeline's Daily Stress Log

Monday

Time: 8 a.m.

Trigger: Train was late, which made me late for work

Response: Angry, frustrated, pressured

Outcome: In the end, I was able to finish proofing the sales report while waiting for the train, and the boss was even later than I was!

Time: 2 p.m.

Trigger: Didn't return an important call because secretary didn't give me a message

Response: Feeling out of control, like a failure

Outcome: The client called back and didn't even realize that I was remiss. I spoke to my secretary and we worked out a more efficient way for her to track incoming calls.

Time: 10 p.m.

Trigger: Getting ready for bed, going over the day in my head

Response: Feeling worried, tense, anxious to solve problems at work

Outcome: I tossed and turned all night, and woke up feeling terrible. I really have to figure this out!

As you can see, the stress triggers in Madeline's life were mostly fairly minor and their results very benign. The one exception was the effect of unrelieved stress on her sleep patterns—because she couldn't deal with her stress at bedtime, Madeline ended up having a very bad night of sleep.

We suggest that you track your stress triggers and responses in the same way, in hopes that you will find a way to better cope with your day-to-day challenges.

Your Daily Stress Log

Time: _____

Trigger: _____

Response: _____

Outcome: _____

Time: _____

Trigger: _____

Response: _____

Outcome: _____

Time: _____

Trigger: _____

Response: _____

Outcome: _____

Time: _____

Trigger: _____

Response: _____

Outcome: _____

Letting Go

Now that you've found out what really bugs you during the day, how can you get rid of the stress that results? Needless to say, one of the most effective ways of reducing stress is to eliminate as many stress-causing agents from your life as possible: changing from your present job to one less fraught with tension, moving to a place more suited to your personality and taste, avoiding people who annoy you, and so on. Unfortunately, making such changes is easier said than done; they'll take some long-range planning and, no doubt, a good deal of self-examination. Not a bad idea, but maybe not so practical when you can't think straight for lack of sleep!

Fortunately, there are several less drastic strategies that you can follow to help relieve your current stress levels. In Chapter 7 we discussed exercise, which is the all-time best way both to alleviate stress and to undo the toll it takes. Here, we outline several other options, ones that use the power of the mind to relax the body.

Biofeedback ABCs

Biofeedback is one of the more scientific methods of revealing and measuring the connection between mind and body—between how you feel and what happens to your body as a result of those feelings. Its underlying premise is that a person can learn to lower his or her heart rate, blood pressure, and other functions of the autonomic nervous system by learning to control the bodily responses involved. In other words, when properly trained, you can learn to lower your blood pressure and slow your heart rate—and thus learn to physiologically, and perhaps emotionally, relax—by concentrating on doing so with your conscious mind.

Biofeedback was developed after studies showed that animals could control their autonomic functions, like blood pressure, when given a reward or punishment. Physicians adapted those findings to design ways for humans to control, through conscious thought, what were once considered unconscious functions. Although there are several biofeedback methods, they all have three things in common:

1. They measure a physiological function (such as blood pressure).
2. They convert this measurement to an understandable form (a blinking light, mercury levels on a thermometer, etc.).
3. They feed back this information to the person.

If you decide to try biofeedback, here's one method you might undergo: You'll be monitored with a machine equipped with lights similar to traffic lights. You'll be fitted with a special blood pressure cuff that has a microphone that will project the sound of any changes in your blood pressure. You'll know if and when your blood pressure starts to rise—one sure sign of stress—because the light on the machine and the sounds emitted from the microphone will let you know. You can then learn to lower your blood pressure by consciously calming down.

Although it sounds very mechanical, biofeedback is, in fact, a process you can learn to master. The ultimate goal is to be able to control your feelings, and their physiological representations, without the machine.

Meditation Made Easy

This is a simple meditation exercise that can help you relax and focus your attention away from the things that cause stress in your life. Start by sitting for just 5 to 10 minutes until you feel comfortable with the practice, then work up to 30 minutes. You may find it helpful to perform your meditation just before going to sleep, but anytime you do it will help reduce overall stress levels. In fact, until you've begun to solve your sleep problem, you may want to avoid practicing this strategy at bedtime when the stakes for relaxing are so high and tension may be the result of a "failed" attempt at meditation.

Basic Meditation Exercise

1. Wear loose, comfortable clothing.

2. Find a quiet place where you won't be disturbed. Turn off the TV or radio, unplug the phone, and ask your family and pets for some privacy.

3. Sit on the floor or bed in a comfortable position. Allow your hands to rest on your legs.

4. Lower your gaze so that your eyes are almost, but not quite, closed.

5. Take a deep breath and let it out slowly.

6. The easiest way to begin meditation is to count your breaths. Inhale, count one. Exhale, count two. Inhale, count three. Repeat the process until you exhale at number ten. Start again, with an inhale, count one.

Breathe Deeply

Another approach to relaxation—and one that's perfect to do in bed as you try to sleep—is deep breathing. When you become distressed, your breathing becomes rapid and shallow. When you're more relaxed, on the other hand, you're probably breathing more slowly and regularly.

Deep Breathing Exercise

1. Get into bed, turn off the lights, and lie flat on your back in a comfortable position.

2. Close your eyes and attempt to concentrate on just your breathing. Leave behind the worries or joys of your day and think only of this moment in time.

3. Visualize your breathing system as consisting of three parts—your abdomen, the middle part near your diaphragm (just beneath your rib cage), and the upper space in your chest. (Please note that only your lungs actually fill with air, but this imagery may help you learn to take deeper, fuller breaths.)

4. As you breathe in through your nose, picture the lower space filling first. Allow your abdomen to expand as air enters the space. Then visualize your middle space filling with energy, light, and air and feel your waistline expand. Feel your chest and your upper back open up as air continues to fill the lungs. The inhalation should take about five seconds.

5. When your lungs feel comfortably full, stop the intake of air.

6. Exhale in a controlled, smooth, continuous movement, the air streaming steadily out of the nostrils. Feel your chest, middle, and stomach gently contract.

   Continue to breathe in this way, concentrating only on your breath. With each inhalation, take in serenity and peace. With each exhalation, let go of worry and physical tension. Before you know it, you'll be asleep.

Progressive Relaxation: On the Road to Sleep

When you can't get to sleep, or when you're worried about something during the day, have you noticed that your forehead wrinkles or your teeth clench, or your hands ball up into a fist? One of the things that happens to your body during times of stress is that your muscles become tense. This occurs because your body is preparing your muscles for action—to fight or to flee a perceived threat to your safety, even if that threat is only a bad night of sleep.

Progressive relaxation is a technique used to induce nerve and muscle relaxation, developed by physician Edmund Jacobsen, for nervous hospitalized patients. The technique involves tensing one muscle group and then relaxing it, slowly moving from one muscle group to another until every muscle group in the body has been affected. As with the meditation and breathing exercises, the idea is to think only of the movement you are making at that moment. This helps you let go of all the worries and stresses of the day.

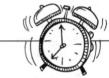

Wake Up!

If you're not used to performing deep breathing exercises, it's especially important to remember to breathe in and out SLOWLY and STEADILY. Otherwise you may hyperventilate and become anxious—just what you want to avoid as you're attempting to relax!

The purpose behind first contracting and then relaxing each muscle is to teach you to recognize more readily what muscle tension feels like. Studies show that relaxing the large skeletal muscles over which you have control can affect the smooth internal muscles over which you normally have no conscious control. As your muscles relax, your blood pressure and heart rate will slow down, and your mind may well stop racing.

Progressive Relaxation Exercise

1. Climb into bed ready to sleep and turn out the lights.
2. Take a deep breath and tighten the muscles of your feet by clenching your toes.
3. As you relax your feet, exhale. Notice the difference in the way your feet feel.
4. Breathe in again, and tighten the muscles of your calves. Hold the exertion for a few seconds. Then exhale and release.
5. Continue the process with your knees, thighs, stomach, chest, arms, shoulders, neck, and face. Each time you tighten and release a muscle group, feel yourself sink deeper and deeper into a state of relaxation. At this point, you should find it much easier to fall asleep.

   As is true for deep breathing or meditation exercises, you should first try performing progressive relaxation at various times during the day instead of only at night. If you're having trouble falling asleep, you may become hyperaware of how the exercise is making you feel instead of allowing it to relax you.

Write Away

If you're the kind of person who goes to bed thinking about everything you didn't get done today, all the things you have to do tomorrow, and what presents you need to buy for Christmas next year, this method of relaxation may be best for you.

Sometime during the evening, at least an hour or two before you go to bed, take out a piece of paper and a pen and find a quiet place to sit. Try to relax and let your mind wander. If you're a worrier—and all you worriers out there know who you are—the things that are bugging you will soon spring to mind. As soon as they do, write them down. They don't have to be important worries and you certainly don't have to find final solutions to them on the spot. Just make sure you write down the thoughts that come to mind during the next 15 or 20 minutes.

When you're finished, take a look at the list. If you like, you can start to sort them into categories such as finances, love life, household chores, etc. Or you can number them in terms of their priority. Then consider solutions or plans of action that might help alleviate the problems you've written down. In this way, you can start to get a handle on the challenges you face.

Then, after you let them sink in, put down the pen, put aside the paper, and promise yourself not to think of what's there until the next day.

You'll be surprised at how much better you'll feel, and that feeling will help you remain relaxed and stress free as you attempt to go to sleep an hour or two later. If a worry creeps back in, you'll know you've written it down along with a potential solution and can thus turn to the important business of falling into a state of deep relaxation and, finally, going to sleep.

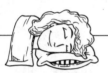

Sleep on it

If possible, leave your worries at the bedroom door. But if you're the type who wakes up with thoughts rushing through your mind, keep a pen and paper handy next to your bed. When a nagging problem wakes you up, write it down. More than likely, you will then be able to put it out of your mind and go back to sleep. Pens with tiny lights attached are available so that you don't have to turn on a bright light—a happy compromise for you and your bed partner!

Don't Worry, Be Sleepy

Before we leave the subject of stress, let's run down the strategies you can employ to relieve the stress that's been keeping you up:

➤ Learn what makes you feel stressed by keeping a daily Stress Log for a week or two.

➤ Exercise.

➤ Practice meditation or other relaxation strategies during the day or just before bed.

➤ Write down your worries before going to bed.

➤ Do NOT stare at the clock.

➤ If you can't sleep, get out of bed, go into another room, and occupy yourself until you feel ready for sleep. Only then return to your bedroom. (We'll talk more about this strategy in Chapter 9.)

With any luck, relieving yourself of excess stress will go a long way toward solving your sleep problem. But the truth is, you'll find it pretty darn hard to fall asleep no matter how relaxed you are if your bedroom is full of light and noise and your mattress strains your neck and back. Read on to find out how to make your bedroom a sanctuary of sleep.

The Least You Need to Know

➤ Stress is an insidious sleep disrupter.

➤ Stress creates a chemical barrier to sleep.

➤ Relaxation strategies work to alleviate the negative effects of stress on the body and the mind.

➤ There are simple steps you can take to ease your body and mind, allowing you to obtain a better night's sleep.

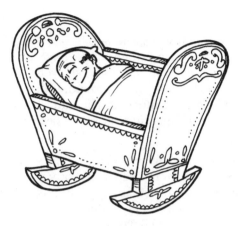

Creating the Right Environment

There's a time and place for everything, as the expression goes—and when it comes to sleep, it's especially true. As this chapter will explain, creating an environment conducive for sleep and developing a regular routine for bedtime may help you solve your current sleep problem—or at the very least, make you more comfortable as you try to get some sleep! First you'll read about the factors in your sleep environment that may be adversely affecting you, then you'll take a quiz that will help you rate the quality of your current sleep environment.

A Sanctuary of Sleep

Ironically enough, the bedroom is often the last place we think to look when searching for a reason for our sleep difficulties. But that's exactly where at least part of the problem may lie.

Take a good look at your bedroom now. Is it free of clutter and distraction? Or is sleeping only one of the many things you do in this room? Does it have window shades that keep out the light? How noisy is it during the night? Is it a "safe zone" in which you can expect a certain amount of privacy and freedom from interruption during your naps and major sleep periods? Let's just see.

Serenity Springs Eternal

It makes sense, doesn't it, that you'd want the room that you sleep in to have a sense of calmness about it, to be free from the ordinary stresses and strains of the day? But if you're like most people, you've got your television plugged in near your bed, your laptop computer on a nearby desk, and the mail piled up on the nightstand. If that sounds like your room, your first priority is to clear away as much of that clutter as you can. Having a serene environment for sleep is one of the first rules of proper sleep hygiene, which we discussed in Chapter 6.

The first thing you should banish from the bedroom is the television set. While some people find that watching a little television helps put them to sleep, many others—especially those already having difficulty falling asleep—are actually quite stimulated by it. Its frantic images, its too-loud commercials, its often anxiety-inducing news reports, and the simple space it takes up in your mind make television an unlikely candidate for the world's "most relaxing activity."

If you find yourself awake and watching television far later than you'd like, then put the set into another room. Watch it there until you feel sleepy, then go back to your bedroom for sleep. Moving the TV out of your bedroom also means that you'll be much less likely to turn it on and then become distracted by it if you awaken in the middle of the night.

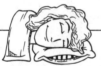

Sleep on it

If you live in a studio apartment, or otherwise simply have no way to separate your work/living space from your sleep space, consider purchasing one or two inexpensive folding screens to place around the potential source of distraction.

As is true for so many sleep solutions, however, you may have to experiment a bit to see if television is a help or a hindrance to your sleep. If you've got a routine that works for you—if hearing Jay Leno's monologue is your sure-fire cue that it's bedtime—then don't mess with it. If not, and you suspect your insomnia may be due to, or exacerbated by, watching too many late, late movies, then remove temptation by removing the television set.

Of course, the TV isn't the only potential source of distraction in your bedroom. Your home computer, a stack of mail, or even just the presence of your briefcase can trigger thoughts of work, bills, and other responsibilities. If you can, clear your nightstand of all but a bedside lamp, an alarm clock (maybe), and perhaps a pleasant vase of your favorite flowers. (We'll get to the issue of clocks in the bedroom a bit later!)

The Light That's Right

If you're like most people, you'll sleep best when it's completely dark in your bedroom. Make sure the hall and bathroom lights are off (or shut the door against them) and cover all windows that get morning light, or light from street lamps and passing cars. Window shades and lined drapes (or a combination of both) are often sufficient for this purpose, but if you're especially sensitive to incoming light, you may want to purchase special blackout shades that totally cover the window surface. Another alternative is wearing eye shades—they not only block out the light but also may lend you a special air of sophistication (remember Audrey Hepburn in *Breakfast at Tiffany's?*).

In Chapter 11, we'll explore the roles of light, circadian rhythms, and sleep in more depth. However, it's important to understand that even the light from a street lamp can disturb your ability to fall or stay asleep—if it's shining directly in your window. You may not even realize how greatly you're disturbed by excess light in the bedroom until you take the time to assess just how much light streams in—from the hallway, bathroom, or outside. Tonight, turn off the lights, allow your eyes to adjust to the darkness, and evaluate how dark (or light) your bedroom really is.

Just for You!

Don't forget that exposure to morning light can help reset your internal biological clock. If you're an Extreme Owl, but you want or need to start getting up and going to bed earlier, then allowing the sun to wake you in the morning may be very helpful.

Quiet, Please!

The plip-plop of a dripping faucet, the sudden scream of an ambulance siren, the thumping bass of a too-loud stereo—any and all of these sounds can prevent or disrupt your sleep. In fact, any unfamiliar sound can wake you up, even if it's an ordinary and not particularly loud noise. On the other hand, over time, you can get used to certain sounds—nearby traffic, the tick of a clock, the chirping of crickets—that might have disturbed you at first.

In addition to light, then, it's also important to monitor your bedroom for sounds that could be disrupting your sleep. If you find that you're exposed to the sound of noisy neighbors, air or street traffic, or other noise while in your bedroom, try using earplugs to shut out all sound. You may also find it helpful to try "white noise"—the sound of an air-conditioner in the summertime, for instance, or the static of a radio set between two stations. You can also try one of the new "environmental sound" machines that play the sounds of the surf or the rain. Many people find these sounds block out disturbing noises and help relax them so they get to sleep.

And, of Course, Sex

A discussion of the sleep environment simply wouldn't be complete without mentioning the one other activity automatically associated with the bed: sex. For most couples, the bed is where it all happens, and it usually happens at night, just before they go to sleep.

The good news is that, for most people, engaging in pleasurable sexual activity at night does not interfere with getting to sleep. In fact, many men and women find that it actually relaxes them and thus helps them to fall asleep even faster than if they'd abstained.

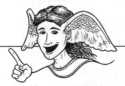

Morpheus Says

Did you know that the act of sexual intercourse involves the release of endorphins, those wonderful brain chemicals that help reduce pain and induce feelings of pleasure? That may be why so many people find that falling asleep after sex is so easy—and why many clinicians believe that sexual activity before sleep may be therapeutic for some people who suffer from sleep-onset insomnia (difficulty in falling, rather than staying, asleep).

On the other hand, the operative word here is *pleasurable*: If sex is stressful or anxiety-provoking for you—and you're having trouble with sleep—you'll only compound your insomnia by relating it in time and space to sexual activity. You should certainly consider seeing your doctor about the problems you're having and, until you've found a way to deal with them, it's probably best to engage in sexual activity outside of the bedroom.

In addition, some people find that having sex stimulates rather than relaxes them. After sex, they remain wide awake—maybe satisfied and happy, but still wide awake!—and often while their partners fall blissfully to sleep. If that sounds like you, you may want to choose to have sex a little earlier in the evenings so that you have a chance to unwind before sleep, or in the mornings so you'll be really ready to roll when the alarm goes off.

Again, the object is to create as uncluttered a bedroom and as serene a bedtime as possible. If having sex helps you fall asleep, then by all means engage! If you find that it disrupts your ability to sleep in any way, then it may be best to find a new time or place.

More Tips for the Weary

In addition to eliminating as many distractions as possible, there are other changes you can make to establish a more serene, calm sleep environment. Here are a few to get you started:

➤ *Hide and mute that tick-tock.* If you're like most people with insomnia, any reminder of the passage of time is a source of stress and anxiety. Put your alarm clock—preferably a digital one that runs silently and is illuminated—inside a dresser drawer. At the very least, turn the clock face from view. The exception to this rule is if you are the kind of person who only gets *more* anxious if you are completely denied access to the clock, in which case, you can simply turn the clock face away from easy view so you avoid "accidentally" looking at it—and becoming tense—in the middle of the night. Again, it's important for you to experiment until you find what works best for you, aiming always for ease, comfort, and relaxation.

➤ *Goldilocks lives!* It's important to keep your bedroom at a comfortable temperature—not too hot or humid and not too cold or dry. For most people, a temperature of about 65 to 68 degrees is about right. Some people like a light breeze from an open window or a ceiling fan, others prefer stillness. Experiment to see what makes you feel best. Again, whatever works for you is appropriate, as long as the practice promotes, rather than interferes with, your ability to sleep.

➤ *Aim for simplicity.* We've already discussed getting rid of anxiety-provoking materials like work files, unpaid bills, unread mail, and the like. But don't forget that pieces of clothing hanging from the furniture, books and magazines piled on a desk, or children's toys littering the floor also may create a feeling of clutter and distraction. Spend just ten minutes tidying up the bedroom before you hit the hay; you may find the act of routine cleaning and the serene environment that results are both sleep promoters.

The Princess and the Pea

Take a moment and fantasize about getting into the "perfect bed." Imagine the feeling that you'll get when you slide between crisp, clean sheets onto a firm but giving mattress, then placing your head on a soft pillow that provides you with just the right amount of head and neck support. And then… and then… just falling into a restful, comfortable sleep.

Now go and get into *your* bed. Does reality match up to the fantasy? Or could your bed and its trappings stand some improvement? Needless to say, if you can't get comfortable in bed, you're going to have a lot more trouble falling asleep.

When Size Matters: The Mattress

Derived from the Arabic *matrah* meaning "to throw down," the first mattresses were probably simple sacks filled with layers of cotton felt. Today, the most popular mattresses sold in the United States—making up more than 80 percent of the market—are innerspring mattresses, which consist of coil springs embedded between layers of upholstery. Other options include futons, waterbeds, foam, and air mattresses.

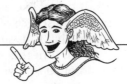

Morpheus Says

Believe it or not, the ancient Egyptians created the first beds—until then most people slept on the ground or on narrow wooden planks. The first beds consisted of crafted wood or other hard material that supported a lattice-work of palm reeds or leather thongs in which people slept. Beds like this were largely reserved for the wealthy classes; Tutankhamen's tomb held a bed made of carved ebony and gold.

If you're one of the vast majority of Americans who own an innerspring mattress, the first question you need to ask yourself when evaluating your current mattress is "Did I buy this before or after Nixon resigned?" Actually, if the answer to that question could even conceivably be "before," you're *way* overdue for a change. The truth is, most mattresses have an average life span of about 10 to 12 years. If you've hit the decade mark, it's time to start thinking about a replacement.

One way to check the health of your mattress is to go to a department store and lie down on a brand new mattress. See how it feels, then go home and try your own. If you notice that your old mattress dips and sags, or if you feel the pinch of sprung springs, chances are you're due for a new one. If so, get yourself back to the store—this time, ready to buy.

When buying a new mattress, there are several factors to consider:

➤ *Size*. Make sure that your bed is large enough to provide ample sleeping space for you. If you're very tall or large, or if you sleep with a partner, then you should consider buying a queen- or even a king-size mattress and bed frame—a full (double) bed is only 54 by 75 inches. A queen-size bed, in comparison, is 60 by 80 inches, and a California king is 72 by 84 inches.

➤ *Firmness*. How firm the mattress should be is definitely a matter of taste as well as physiology. A mattress should support your lower back and keep your spine in alignment from its base to your head. If you suffer from arthritis or another condition that causes joint or muscle pain, you probably will feel better on a firmer rather than softer mattress.

➤ *Cost*. Generally speaking, the more you pay, the better mattress you'll get. That said, there is a wide range of prices for satisfactory products, starting at the lower end—about $300—and going all the way up to $1,200 and more. The best advice: Spend as much as you can, and your body will thank you for it.

Pillow Talk

Believe it or not, your head accounts for a full 20 percent of your body weight and, therefore, needs to be well supported when you're lying down. Down or feather pillows are usually best (except in the case of allergies, which we discuss below) because they "give" better than polyester fills, which can be stiff and inflexible.

Your pillow should support the head and neck, keeping them in alignment with the spine—no matter what sleeping position you take. Generally speaking, you'll want a firmer pillow if you sleep on your side, a medium-firm pillow if you sleep on your back, and a soft pillow if you sleep on your stomach.

Taking the Right Position

Back sleepers, side sleepers, stomach sleepers, tossers and turners...everyone has his or her favorite sleep style. How you sleep best is the position you want to be in—as long as you also feel comfortable during the day. If you sleep on your stomach and wake with lower back pain, you may want to try adjusting to a side position (some people find that stacking pillows in front and behind them will help them maintain this position). If you sleep on your back and your partner tells you that you snore, a side position may also help solve this problem.

When all is said and done, however, even the best bedroom environment will do nothing to help a very awake, overstimulated person get to sleep. If you find yourself all wound up with no place to go when it's time for bed, then you may need to re-evaluate how you spend your evening hours.

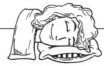

Sleep on it

If you're pregnant, many experts advice that you use two pillows, one upon which to rest your head and the other to place between your knees as you sleep on your side. This position is best because it prevents you from sleeping on your back, a position that puts all the weight on a major blood vessel (the inferior vena cava), as well as strains back muscles.

Wake Up!

If you suffer from allergies, be sure to identify and remove potential allergens from the bedroom. Choose bedclothes and pillows with care, remove all rugs (which can become depositories for dust mites, pollen, dander, and other airborne allergens), and consider getting an air-conditioner fitted with a special air filter to keep you breathing easily throughout the night.

A Nighttime Ritual Just for You

The hour or so before you go to bed is extremely important in setting the stage for an easy descent into sleep. You can make this time work for you by following a regular, restful routine. Here are some tips:

➤ *Avoid stimulation.* About an hour before you want to fall asleep, put away the mail, stop writing down your worries (as described in Chapter 8), and simply try to relax.

➤ *Ease off.* Many people find that performing a few easy, slow stretches helps get the kinks out of the body and puts the mind in the mood for sleep. If you decide to make stretching a part of your pre-bedtime routine, do not overexert yourself or stimulate your muscles. Relax into the stretches and never push.

➤ *Heat up.* A warm bath, preferably one scented with an oil like lavender—known for its calming attributes—is another relaxing ritual that helps set the stage for sleep. In addition to soothing body and soul, a warm bath also raises body temperature; cooling down afterwards is one of the triggers for sleep.

➤ *Stick to the plan.* As we've tried to make clear in this and previous chapters, when it comes to sleeping well the most important thing about your nighttime experience is setting up a routine that works for you—then sticking to it. Your body's internal clock easily becomes disrupted when unexpected changes occur. If sipping a glass of herbal tea while you take a warm bath provides you with a restful night's sleep, then perform that ritual as often as you can and at as regular a time as possible.

And So to Bed

After reading this chapter, how would you rate your sleep environment and bedtime routine? Take this quiz and see:

Your Sleep Hygiene Quiz

Circle the number that best describes your situation.

1. My room is free from loud or sudden noises.

   Poor   **Excellent**

   1   2   3   4   5

2. I sleep in darkness, using window shades or eye covers if necessary.

   Poor   **Excellent**

   1   2   3   4   5

3. My room temperature is comfortable and allows me to sleep well.

   Poor   **Excellent**

   1   2   3   4   5

4. My mattress and pillow are firm enough to support me and soft enough to offer comfort.

   Poor   **Excellent**

   1   2   3   4   5

5. I have enough fresh air in my bedroom.

   Poor   **Excellent**
   1   2   3   4   5

6. I perform regular, relaxing activities (e.g., warm bath, easy stretches, etc.) during the hour or two before I go to bed each night.

   Poor   **Excellent**
   1   2   3   4   5

Score the quiz by adding up the numbers you've circled. If your total score is between 25 and 30, you've designed your bedroom well and have established a nighttime ritual that works for you. If you suffer from insomnia and score between 20 and 25, look at the questions you've circled with a "2" or "1" and start making changes there. If you score 20 or less, your bedroom definitely needs some work. Take another look at some of the tips we've offered here, and see if you can improve your sleep by touching up your sleep environment.

Next, we'll tackle what can be a touchy subject: the use of prescription medication, over-the-counter remedies, and herbal potions to improve sleep. In Chapter 10, we'll outline the risks and benefits of these substances so that you can make an informed choice about what's right for you.

The Least You Need to Know

➤ Your sleep environment is an important factor when it comes to getting a good night's sleep.

➤ You're likely to improve the quality of your sleep by purchasing a proper mattress and pillow.

➤ Maintaining a relaxing pre-bedtime routine will help you feel more relaxed and ready for sleep.

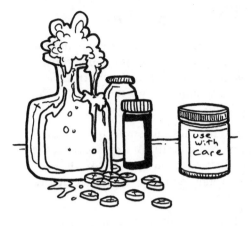

Chapter 10

Sleeping Pills and Potions

In This Chapter

➤ When sleeping pills and potions might help

➤ The power of narcotics

➤ Understanding the role of melatonin and tryptophan

➤ Exploring herbal remedies

To someone struggling with chronic insomnia, it's often too tempting to resist the quick-fix approach to getting rid of anxiety and exhaustion so that sleep—deep, restful sleep—is possible. That's why "sleep cures" of all kinds—from prescription medications to over-the-counter remedies to herbal supplements—remain so popular. According to a 1990 estimate by the National Sleep Foundation, consumers spend more than $1.1 billion a year on products used to promote sleep.

But like most other ideas that sound too good to be true, these quick fixes usually fail to achieve your ultimate goal—improving your sleep over the long term. By taking any substance to help you sleep, you're treating only the symptom, not the underlying problem. Until you figure out what's really keeping you from getting a good night's sleep, and solving it from that perspective, you'll still have a sleep problem when you wake up the next day.

That said, there is a time and place for such sleep aids. And, if you take them as directed and with care, you may be able to get the rest you need without suffering any adverse effects. In this chapter, we'll help you sort out the myths from the facts about sleeping pills and over-the-counter potions so that you can make a more informed decision about what's right for you.

Sleeping Pills, the Brain, and Your Body

According to recent research, more than 13 million people in the United States take some kind of prescribed medication to improve their sleep. A sleeping pill is any medication used to promote sleep and treat insomnia. As we'll discuss further in a moment, there are several types of sleeping pills available today, each one affecting the brain and body in a different way.

In general, sleeping pills act to sedate and depress the arousal centers in the brain, thereby promoting sleep (and often reducing anxiety as well). To a greater or lesser degree, depending on their make-up, sleeping pills reduce the time it takes to reach sleep onset, make it easier to fall asleep, increase total sleep time, and decrease the number of awakenings.

Night Owl Wisdom

Rebound insomnia is a common side effect that occurs after sleeping pill use is terminated, and the insomnia comes back—sometimes with even more stubbornness. REM sleep is also disturbed, and some people also report having terrible nightmares.

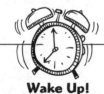

Wake Up!

Never stop taking prescription medication without first discussing the matter with your physician. You may need to taper off your use of the drug in order to prevent suffering serious side effects and withdrawal symptoms.

However—and this is a big however—all sleeping pills also have significant drawbacks when it comes to long-term, or even medium-term, use. These drawbacks include:

➤ *Sleep quality.* Most sleeping pills alter your sleep architecture, increasing the amount of time you spend in lighter Stage 2 sleep and decreasing the time you spend in deep Stages 3 and 4 and REM sleep. This means that your brain and body do not receive the full recovery benefits of natural sleep on the nights you take a sleeping aid.

➤ *Dependence.* Taking sleeping pills may create a vicious circle of dependence: Most pills work well only for a relatively short amount of time—a few weeks or months at most. After that, two things can happen: You not only can become dependent on them, but also may have to up the dosage bit by bit or change medications often in order to reap any benefit. Or you can quit them altogether. In some cases, especially if you only used sleeping pills for a brief period to get yourself through a bad time, you'll be just fine. If, on the other hand, you've used sleeping pills for a longer period of time than suggested, or if you're particularly sensitive to the medication, you may develop another problem: *rebound insomnia*.

➤ *Rebound insomnia.* The really miserable thing about overusing sleeping pills is that once you decide to stop, your problem with sleep may only become worse. For reasons not yet completely understood, withdrawing from sleeping pills—

sometimes after taking them just a few times—brings back the original insomnia, often with a greater intensity. And this rebound effect can last up to several weeks.

➤ *Side effects.* Daytime sleepiness, temporary memory loss, confusion, dizziness, weakness, nausea, delayed reaction time, loss of appetite, and frequent urination are some of the many side effects caused by most sleeping pills. Among the most dangerous (as you might suspect) are those that affect your ability to function the next day. Accidents of all kinds are more likely to occur if you are not alert and are unable to react. As is true for the drugs' effects, side effects also vary from individual to individual, with some very sensitive people having strong reactions while others experience few or no problems at all.

➤ *Risk of interactions.* The active ingredients in sleeping pills can counteract or, conversely, enhance the effects of other medications and alcohol. As central nervous system depressants, they act to slow down respiration and the heart rate as do alcohol, antihistamines, and other medications. If you take too much of these central nervous system depressants, the effects can be deadly. Medication used to promote sleep can also interfere with the metabolism of other medications. Therefore, your doctor may need to adjust the dosage appropriately. NEVER DRINK ALCOHOL when you're taking a sleep medication. The result could be lethal.

Wake Up!

A side effect of most sleeping pills is a slowdown in respiration, which makes breathing more difficult. For people with respiratory problems, heart problems, or sleep apnea, a depressed respiratory system can be deadly. Discuss all possible risks and side effects with your doctor *before* taking any medication.

The Doctor's Cabinet: Prescription Sleep Aids

When choosing a sleeping medication that's right for you, your doctor will take a wide variety of factors into consideration, including your symptoms, what he or she knows about your physiological makeup, other medications you're taking, and the action of the specific drug itself. Among the general choices your doctor has are the following classes of drugs; within these classes are literally dozens of different medications:

➤ *Benzodiazepines.* Now the most common prescription drugs for insomnia, benzodiazepines induce sleep by suppressing arousal centers in the brain. Compared to older sleeping pills (see below), they have relatively few side effects and drug interactions. Some benzodiapines (such as triazalam [Halcion]) are short-acting, while others (such as flurazepam [Dalmane]) are long-acting, which can make you feel sleepy during the day. You can become dependent on any of these medications in a relatively short time, however, and they should be used only under the careful direction of a physician.

119

➤ *Barbiturates*. Barbiturates are sedatives; that is, they act to depress the central nervous system. Not only do they suppress the arousal centers in the brain (helping you to sleep), they also affect the heart rate, decrease the blood pressure, and lower body temperature. Because of the wide range of effects and side effects, doctors today almost never prescribe barbiturates to new users, and often advise current users to switch to newer medication. Only in rare cases are barbiturates used to treat insomnia.

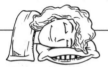

Sleep on it

If you're finding it impossible to sleep because you're facing a particularly difficult emotional or physical challenge, talk to your doctor. Taking a sleeping pill for a few nights may help you regain your strength and prevent insomnia from becoming yet another stressful problem for you to solve.

Night Owl Wisdom

The **half-life** of a medication is the length of time it takes for your body to break the drug down into inactive forms or to eliminate it. A drug with a short half-life may be out of your body completely after 5 hours or so, while longer-acting ones may continue to have an effect for 24 hours or more.

➤ *Imidazopyridines*. This new class of drugs, of which only one is now available—under the brand name Ambien (zolpidem)—appears to be far safer than barbiturates and poses even lower risks of side effects, drug interactions, rebound insomnia, and addiction than benzodiazepines. Another benefit of zolpidem is that it does not appear to reduce the time spent in deep and REM sleep stages, one of the biggest drawbacks of some other medications.

➤ *Sedating antidepressants*. Another option for those suffering from insomnia is an antidepressant that also acts as a sedative. Even if you don't also suffer from depression, you might benefit from this treatment if you've experienced side effects from other types of sleeping medication, have a history of alcohol or drug dependence, or have a medical condition that precludes the use of a central nervous system depressant. Antidepressants also pose little risk of dependence. Unfortunately, they, too, have their potential side effects, including changes in heart rate, dry mouth, urine retention, and impairment in sexual function.

➤ *Antihistamines*. As anyone who's taken an antihistamine to treat allergies can tell you, this type of medication does more than clear up your sinuses and reduce itching. In most people, certain antihistamines also have a sedating effect that, if timed properly, can help reduce the time it takes to reach sleep onset at night. However, not all antihistamines help to sedate (some actually act as stimulants) and most work only for a night or two at best. Antihistamines can also have significant side effects, including dizziness, gastric distress, dryness of the mouth and nose, and disturbed coordination. You can buy some antihistamines over the counter, while others are by prescription only.

Among the most important qualities of a sleeping medication is its uptake (the time needed for it to take effect) and its *half-life*, (the time needed for your body to break down and eliminate it). Some medications work very quickly, which means you should take them just before or as you go to bed—and these medications may be helpful if middle-of-the-night awakenings are a problem for you. It's important to know the half-life of a drug because that determines how long the average person will feel its effects; some medications are out of your body quickly, whereas others affect you for far longer than you might desire.

Despite the risks of taking medication to help you sleep, we want to state clearly once again that there *are* circumstances that warrant it. The most important thing you can do for your health is to discuss the matter thoroughly with your doctor before taking any medication for this purpose.

You and Your Doctor

Insomnia is one of those symptoms for which there is no objective clinical evidence. That means that your doctor must depend on your subjective description of your own symptoms in order to make a decision about your need for a sleeping aid. It's up to you to be as open and honest as possible about your problem. If your sleep problem is more than a temporary side effect of a brief emotional upset or physical illness, you'll still have a sleep problem when you wake up after taking sleeping pills.

When used appropriately, however, prescription medications can be both effective and safe. Generally, prescription sleep medications are limited to short-term use (7 to 10 days), after which you'll need to see your doctor again for a re-evaluation. There are several questions to ask your doctor if he or she prescribes a sleep medication for you:

➤ Why do you recommend this drug?

➤ How does the drug act to alleviate symptoms?

➤ What are the possible side effects?

➤ Will the drug interact with other medications I'm taking?

➤ What is the recommended schedule and dosage?

➤ Should I avoid alcohol while taking this medication?

➤ How long should I take it?

➤ What other steps can I take to solve my sleep problem?

By discussing the answers to these questions with your doctor, both of you can make an informed decision about which, if any, medication is right for your needs. You and your doctor should meet regularly to evaluate the effects and side effects of any medication you decide to take and to monitor the progress of your sleep problem.

Although it's especially important to be aware of the actions and side effects of prescription medications, there are almost as many precautions to take when it comes to over-the-counter sleep aids (OTCs).

Over-the-Counter and Through the Wood

The National Sleep Foundation estimates that about 40 percent of individuals suffering from insomnia self-medicate with OTCs or alcohol to hasten sleep. OTCs usually contain antihistamines that cause the same heavy-headed drowsiness that many cold medicines do.

Wake Up!

Just like prescription medications, over-the-counter remedies can interact with other medications you may be taking. If you take another medication, please talk to your doctor before taking an OTC formula.

As discussed, antihistamines can also cause side effects, including dry mouth and dry eyes. If you take a large dose, or are particularly sensitive, sleepiness and even disorientation can last well into the next day.

It's important to be aware that side effects can creep up on you even with OTC medications. You may not realize how drowsy or disoriented you feel until you find yourself trying to cross the street against the light or attempting to sharpen a ball-point pen in the pencil sharpener. If you decide to take an OTC, pay special attention to how you feel the next day. If side effects are limited, and you experience only very occasional bouts of insomnia, then feel free to partake. If you find yourself using a product more than once a week, however, talk to your doctor about the trouble you're having with sleep. Clearly, you'll need to address the underlying problem before you'll find a permanent solution.

Melatonin and Tryptophan: Myths or Miracles?

Melatonin and tryptophan are two substances produced in the body that are known for their sleep-promoting properties. However, the scientific literature offers a mixed assessment of melatonin's effectiveness and potential risks. And the history of tryptophan's use offers additional cautions.

Since neither melatonin nor tryptophan are legally considered drugs, they have not had to undergo the same kind of laboratory and clinical testing as substances considered medications. The Federal Drug Administration (FDA) does not have jurisdiction over naturally occurring substances, such as vitamins, amino acids, herbs, and hormones (like melatonin)—as long as their manufacturers make no health claims about them. If the manufacturers claim that melatonin is a "sleep aid," for instance, the FDA can consider it to be a drug and thus subject to the same strict rules and regulations used for prescription pharmaceuticals.

So far, however, melatonin, tryptophan, and most herbs (which we'll discuss later) remain outside the agency's purview. As a consumer, then, you need to conduct as much research about these products as you can by reading books like this one, talking to your doctor, and monitoring news reports about new studies conducted on these substances.

Melatonin: The "Dark" Hormone

Melatonin is a substance produced by the body's pineal gland, which lies at the base of the brain. Known as the "chemical expression of darkness," melatonin is produced almost exclusively during the night, when it is dark. In healthy young adults, melatonin levels are lowest during the day, increase during the evening hours, and peak in the middle of the night.

As mentioned in Chapter 2, melatonin plays an important role in organizing daily circadian rhythms. High levels of the hormone send a biological signal to the brain to begin nighttime behavior, and decreasing levels signal the onset of daytime activity. As you get older, the amount of melatonin you produce diminishes, primarily because the pineal gland shrinks and calcifies with age. Some research indicates that one of the reasons older people have trouble staying asleep during the night is that they produce low levels of melatonin.

The theory behind using melatonin supplements—capsules, tablets, or liquids created in a laboratory—as a sleep aid is twofold: First, taking melatonin may help reset the body's clock by triggering the sleep response in the brain at a different time than it would normally occur. For this reason, many people find that taking melatonin helps them adjust to a new time zone more quickly than they would otherwise. Second, melatonin is also a sleep promoter; that is, a dose of melatonin before bedtime acts as a relatively immediate sleep aid in some people who take it—and, for most people, without any short-term side effects. (Since widespread use of melatonin supplements is relatively recent, a thorough exploration of its potential long-term side effects has not been completed.)

Unfortunately, researchers remain divided on what effects taking melatonin supplements really has on either disturbed biological rhythms or insomnia. There appears to be more evidence in favor of its use for jet lag, sleep/wake rhythm disorders (see Chapter 14), and for night-shift workers than for chronic insomnia.

It remains unclear what, if any, dose of melatonin is best, when doses should be administered, and to whom. In fact, that's what makes it so tricky: Some people find that melatonin helps them fall asleep and stay asleep, while others experience no effect, and still others find it makes them feel groggy the next day—a hazardous side effect if there ever was one. Some people even report that melatonin causes them to feel too agitated and anxious to sleep.

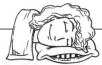

Sleep on it

Many melatonin supplements currently on the market come in tablets of up to 3 mgs—over 10 times more than you need to reset your biological clock or to feel sleepy. We suggest that you buy brands that come in 1 mg doses and cut the tablet in half, and perhaps even into thirds, so that you take only 0.5 or 0.3 mg per night.

Currently, melatonin supplements are available in various dosages—usually from 1 to 3 milligrams—in tablet or liquid form, which is more than your body produces in a day. Recent research suggests that you need far less than even the smallest dose to obtain results: Only 0.3 milligram or a third of the 1 milligram dose. Although melatonin supplements appear to be perfectly safe for most people in the short term, it's important to understand that melatonin is a powerful hormone, and even in small doses, it may affect a number of different body processes.

You should NOT take melatonin if you:

➤ Are pregnant, trying to get pregnant, or breast-feeding

➤ Suffer from an autoimmune disease, diabetes, epilepsy, leukemia, or migraine headaches

➤ Are taking cortisone medication

➤ Are coping with kidney disease

And, as we've said before, talk to your doctor before taking any sleeping aid.

Tryptophan

Studies of tryptophan's effects on sleep offer mixed results. According to Peter Hauri in his excellent book *No More Sleepless Nights* (Wiley, 1990), there are at least 25 studies suggesting that taking tryptophan supplements in the evening helps about half of all insomniacs—and that sometimes the supplements are even more effective than prescription medications. Other studies, however, show no such benefit.

To complicate matters, in 1988 and 1989 more than 1,500 people fell ill and 35 people died from a rare disorder called Eosinophilia Myalgia Syndrome, and their only common link was that they all used tryptophan to help them sleep. It appears that just one batch of tryptophan may have been contaminated during the manufacturing process and caused the syndrome to develop in those who took it. Nevertheless, this incident caused many doctors and patients alike to be wary of recommending and using tryptophan supplements.

If you want to see whether tryptophan will work for you, we recommend you try getting a dose of it from the foods you eat. As you may remember from Chapter 7, tryptophan is found in milk, meat, fish, eggs, and peanuts, so a glass of warm milk may do you as much good as taking a tryptophan supplement—and at far less risk.

The Herbal Route

In 1992, the U.S. National Institutes of Health, the federal government's largest supporter of medical research, announced the establishment of the Office of Alternative Medicine. Its goal remains to explore approaches to such chronic diseases as allergies, arthritis, heart disease—and, yes, insomnia—for which conventional Western medicine offers limited treatment options.

Among the most popular alternatives—and the one under a great deal of scrutiny by modern Western scientists—is the use of plants and plant material as medicine. Echinacea for colds, ginseng for anxiety and other conditions, and ginkgo biloba for Alzheimer's disease are just a few of the remedies that fall under the rubric of "herbal medicine."

Herbs as Medicine

The use of herbs has been integral to the practice of medicine since the beginning of human society. In fact, the word *drug* comes from the old Dutch word *drogge*, meaning "to dry," as pharmacists, physicians, and ancient healers often dried plants for use as medicines. Today, approximately 25 percent of all prescription drugs are still derived from trees, shrubs, or herbs. Interestingly enough, the World Health Organization noted in 1985 that of 119 plant-derived pharmaceutical medicines, about 74 percent are used in modern medicine in ways that correlate directly with their traditional uses as plant medicines.

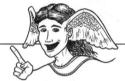

Morpheus Says

To date, only about 5,000 of the estimated 250,000 to 500,000 plant species have been extensively studied for their medicinal applications, which means we may yet hear of new plant-based remedies in the future. In the meantime, it's important to remember that herbs *are* medicines that may have risks and side effects.

Generally speaking, herbal medicines work in much the same way as do conventional pharmaceutical drugs. Herbs contain a large number of naturally occurring substances that work to alter the body's chemistry so it can return it to its natural state of health. Unlike manufactured drugs, however, plants and other organic materials contain a wide variety of substances and, hence, less of any one particular active alkaloid. Herbs are thus less likely to be toxic to the body than are most pharmaceutical products.

On the other hand, it's important to stress that herbs have only recently come under intense medical study, and thus we have few data on which to base either their effectiveness or their safety. Because the use of natural herbs has not come under the scrutiny of Western medicine for very long—and because many physicians have little experience using them with patients—definitive research about their benefits is relatively sparse. The good news is that, for most people, the risk of developing side effects from normal use is very small. Nevertheless, again, we want to stress caution when it comes to taking any substance—talk to your doctor before doing so.

Herbs for Insomnia

There are several herbs thought to help relax the body and induce sleep. Some are brewed to make teas, others are used as essential oils in the bath or dabbed on pillowcases. As discussed, however, the FDA does not regulate herbs—like vitamins, minerals, and other supplements, herbs are not treated as drugs. That means that you can't be absolutely sure of the strength, quality, or effectiveness of the products you buy. Seeking the help of a licensed practitioner of natural medicine or herbalist may help answer any questions you may have.

Before you read about the herbs useful for sleep, it's important to stress that in addition to any medicinal properties of the herbs themselves, you'll benefit from the ritual of preparation. Simply making a cup of warm tea or a warm bath part of your nightly ritual will aid you in your journey toward regular, restful sleep.

Among the most popular herbal remedies for insomnia are:

➤ *Chamomile* (Anthriscus cerefolium). Chamomile is used both as a tea and as a medicinal herb. You can buy chamomile tea in almost every grocery store, and you can buy chamomile flowers and leaves by mail order to make your own remedies. Some people claim that sleeping on a pillow stuffed with chamomile flowers, for example, makes for a particularly restful night's sleep.

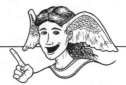

Morpheus Says

The early Egyptians dedicated the chamomile plant to the Sun God because of its fever-reducing effects. And Pliny, the early Roman scholar, recommended baths of chamomile to treat headaches and kidney disorders. We now use it to both relax the nervous system—making it a helpful sleep promoter—and to soothe the digestive system.

➤ *Hops* (Humulus lupulus). Hops has been used as a flavoring and preservative in beer since the 9th century, and has had an even longer history as an herbal remedy for insomnia. The active ingredient in hops is lupulnic acid, which suppresses central nervous system activity and helps induce sleep. Hops is available in commercial herbal remedies as dried or fresh herbs from which to make a tea and in the form of capsules, powder, and *tinctures*. You can add drops of the tincture into boiling water and drink it like a tea.

➤ *Lavender* (Lavandula officinalis). The fragrance of this plant is most often associated with lace sachets and hand soap. However, the true scent of lavender has a clean, fresh quality about it, which perhaps motivated the Romans to name it after *lavare*, meaning "to wash." Lavender is available as a tea, tincture, or aromatic essential oil.

➤ *Passionflower* (Passiflora incarnata). Often used in Europe as a mild, hypnotic, sedative herb to calm the nervous system and promote sleep, passionflower is also known as maypop, a woody vine that flowers in the spring. It contains low levels of serotonin, which may help explain the use of the plant as a natural sedative. It comes in capsule form.

➤ *Valerian* (Valerian officinalis). Quaintly known as the "Valium of the 19th century," valerian is widely recognized for its relaxing effect on the body. In Europe, doctors often prescribe it to treat anxiety. Its medicinal qualities are found in the root of the plant, which has a disagreeable odor. Fortunately, valerian is available as a pill or capsule, as well as a tincture. Most people prefer to take the pill because the roots have a bitter taste.

Now that you've read about some of the pharmaceutical and herbal remedies for sleep, it's time to look at one of the most obvious yet largely unappreciated influences on our sleep/wake patterns: light. In Chapter 11, we'll show you how to make light your very best friend when it comes to setting and maintaining healthy, steady biological rhythms.

Night Owl Wisdom

A **tincture** is a preparation made by soaking flowers, leaves, roots, or other parts of plant material in a solution of alcohol. Health food stores and herbalists sell tinctures already prepared, or can offer you the materials you need to make one yourself.

Wake Up!

Talk to an experienced herbalist before taking any herbs. Although herbs generally act gently on your body, they can cause side effects if taken in high doses or if you're particularly sensitive to them. Both hops and passionflower, for instance, can exacerbate depression in some people. Pay attention to how you react when you try a new remedy for any reason.

The Least You Need to Know

➤ There are appropriate times to take a sleeping pill or potion.

➤ Taking prescription medication requires vigilance on your part and the close scrutiny of a medical professional.

➤ Over-the-counter sleep aids may be helpful, but they, too, have their risks and side effects.

➤ There may be a role for melatonin and tryptophan supplements, but you should use caution if you decide to take them.

➤ Herbal remedies may be safer than—and they're possibly just as effective as—pharmaceuticals, though you still need to use caution should you decide to take them.

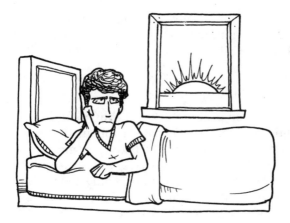

Chapter 11

Let There Be Light

In This Chapter

➤ Understanding the power of light

➤ Exploring the connection between light and mood

➤ Gathering light from new technology

Light: It's a "utility" most of us take for granted, but it's also a crucial topic when it comes to any discussion of a good night's sleep. Indeed, the amount of light to which you're exposed, how bright that light is, and at what time of the day you receive it, play important roles in controlling your circadian rhythms. As you'll see later, gaining an understanding of how light affects you is especially important if you work the night shift or have difficulty adjusting to time-zone travel, but almost everyone is affected, for better or worse, by their exposure (or lack of it) to light.

The path of sunlight across the surface of our spinning planet, with its regular progression of sunrises and sunsets, and our planet's revolution around the sun determined much of our ancestors' day-to-day and seasonal lives, from when they got up in the morning to when they planted their crops. These days, most of us frequently become disconnected from the natural rhythms set by our strongest and most essential Zeitgeber—the sun—which could be one reason why so many people have sleep problems. Most people in modern, industrial societies receive too much of the wrong kind of light (primarily dim, artificial light) and too little of the right kind (full-spectrum bright natural daylight). Because of this, we inadvertently play havoc with our internal circadian clocks, thereby disrupting our sleep, our moods, and other aspects of our physical and mental health.

Learning about the potential effects of light on your sleep/wake patterns will help you better manipulate your exposure to it in order to improve your sleep at night and alertness levels during the day. In this chapter, we'll show you how to do just that.

Light and Your Brain

The intensity of the light falling on us is measured in *lux*, which is the international unit of illumination. When you're standing outside, you're exposed to about 10,000 lux on a heavy, overcast day; 50,000 lux on a sunny day; and 100,000 lux or more on an open beach or snow-covered ground where much light is reflected from the surface. Indoor light from incandescent or fluorescent light bulbs may provide only 200 to 500 lux depending on how far you are from the light. Many industrial workplaces provide even less light at night. In such places, light levels of 5 to 50 lux—or even less—are common. People who work at computer stations controlling oil refineries or nuclear power stations, for instance, may receive less than 5 lux.

The amount of light to which you're exposed varies considerably depending on where you are and what kind of day it is: Outside on a sunny day, you receive from 5 to 10 times as much light as you do on a cloudy day— and more than 100 times as much as you do in the average indoor office.

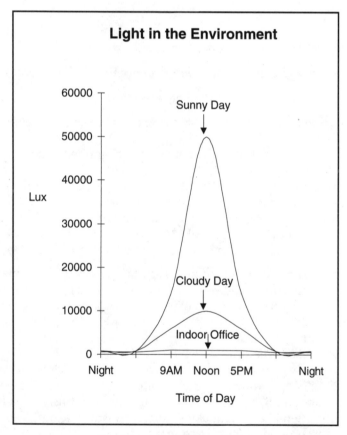

Copyright © 1998 by Circadian Information Limited Partnership. Reprinted with permission. All rights reserved.

The primary way the brain receives light is through the eyes, though recent research indicates that other body cells (including, perhaps, blood cells) are also sensitive to light. Light sends a signal that is conveyed to that tiny group of brain cells called the suprachiasmatic nuclei (SCN). As we mentioned earlier, these cells appear to be the master internal clock that drives the body's sleep/wake and other biological patterns. As discussed in Chapter 2, light in the morning and darkness at night are the two most important cues that keep these rhythms in synch. Without regular and well-timed exposure to the natural cycles of light and darkness, you may well end up with a sleep problem.

Understanding the Timing of Light

When it comes to how light affects your biological rhythms, you must consider not only how bright the light is, but also when you're exposed to it. Indeed, the effect that light has on your circadian rhythms depends to a large degree on what time of day or night you are exposed to it.

Night Owl Wisdom

Lux is the metric unit used to quantify the intensity of visible light. (1 lux is approximately equal to 11 footcandles.) It represents the amount of light that eventually falls upon an object or a person from a source—not necessarily the amount of light being emitted from that source. On a cloudy day, 10,000 lux reach you from the sky, whereas you're suffused by more than 50,000 lux from the sun when the skies are blue.

As we've discussed, light is the primary Zeitgeber, the cue that helps maintain your daily rhythms by signaling the time of day to the brain. Therefore, depending on what point in the day or night exposure to bright light occurs, you can either advance or delay your circadian rhythms. Your body clock's reaction to light falls on a continuum, called the phase response curve (PRC). The PRC describes the number of hours of shift in the setting of the biological clock that occurs when an individual is exposed to bright light.

During the day, your biological clock virtually ignores light signals, since that's when it naturally expects sunlight to fall. At night, between the hours of 10 p.m. to 5 a.m., however, exposure to sufficiently bright light acts to delay the timing of the clock, in effect shifting it westward. The later and the more intense this exposure is, the greater the shift westward. Exposure to light from 5 a.m. to 8 a.m., on the other hand, nudges the biological clock eastward. The strongest shifts westward or eastward occur when exposure to light takes place closest to the "breakpoint" of about 5 a.m., or about two hours before normal wake-up time, which is near your body temperature minimum.

As this graphic shows, exposure to light may shift your body clock backward or forward, or have no effect on it at all, depending on what time of day or night the exposure occurs. During daylight hours (represented by the dots), no shift occurs with light exposure. At night the closer you get to the breakpoint (typically about 5 a.m.), the more your biological clock will shift in response to light. Before the breakpoint, the shift results in a "westbound delay," which means you'll naturally stay up later and get up later. After the breakpoint, bright light exposure forces an "eastward advance," which means you'll naturally go to bed earlier and get up earlier. Learning to manipulate your exposure to bright light can help you more quickly adjust to time-zone changes and shift work.

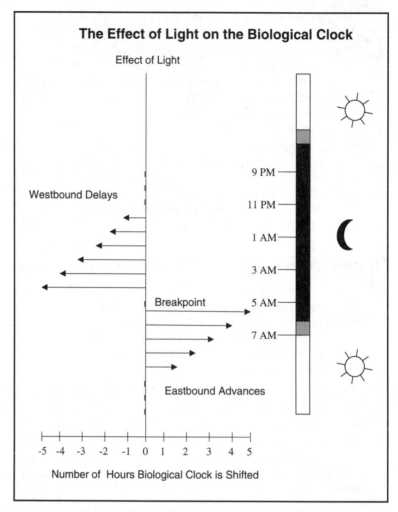

The Effect of Light on the Biological Clock

Armed with this knowledge, it is possible for you to set your biological clock to any time zone on the planet—provided you adequately control your exposure to light and dark. Using dark sunglasses, keeping skin surfaces covered, staying indoors, and blackening the bedroom windows can give you control of your exposure to darkness. Going out in the daylight or sunlight, or using artificial bright light sources can give you the necessary exposure to light.

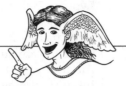

Morpheus Says

Although bright light intensities of 2,500 lux or greater are necessary to shift your body clock by an hour or more in one shot, if you expose yourself to smaller amounts—even as little as 200 to 500 lux—every day at the same time for 4 or 5 days, you may gradually nudge the biological clock and eventually achieve an equal shift forward or backward. Even reading in bed for a few hours after 11 p.m., night after night, might help to reset your biological clock, making it increasingly difficult to go to sleep at an earlier time after a week or so.

Let's say you're jetting off from Boston to Paris and want to know how to best avoid jet lag by resetting your clock. When do you need exposure to light? If you're like most travelers, you'll get off the plane at 7 a.m. local time—but at 1 a.m. body time. Light in the early Paris morning will reset your clock toward Hawaii time—in the totally wrong direction. Instead of taking a stroll outside, keep your sunglasses on until you reach your hotel, stay in the darkness (napping if you like) until about 11 a.m., then go outside and sit in the sun. A precisely timed exposure to the light from 11 a.m. to 1 p.m. will help you adapt to the local scene much more quickly than you otherwise would. We'll discuss this further in Chapter 18.

Providing light in the right amounts at the right time to help you solve your sleep problems—whether they're caused by a sleep disorder, time-zone travel, or night-shift work—is tricky business, one better left to sleep specialists. However, you can see that bright light exposure is an important factor in your sleep/wake patterns. Depending on your climate, or on your individual needs, finding the right light may be a challenge.

Light Up Your Life

In addition to helping set and maintain your body's internal clock, light also enhances your alertness. Both bright and moderate light cause you to become more awake and alert than you might otherwise be. In laboratory studies at the Institute for Circadian Physiology, for instance, people who were exposed to 1,000 lux during simulated night shifts were less likely to fall asleep on the job, and they also scored better on cognitive performance tests than workers left in the relative dark.

Exactly why light enhances alertness is not well understood. The leading theory is that light suppresses the brain's production of melatonin, a hormone that promotes sleepiness. Some studies also indicate that exposure to light raises body temperature, which helps boost alertness and mental performance.

Night Owl Wisdom

Seasonal Affective Disorder, also known as **SAD**, is a recurrent mood disorder characterized by depressive episodes and related symptoms that develop during the fall and winter and often remit when the seasons pass.

As you can see, light significantly affects when you wake, when you sleep, and how you feel—a point we'll discuss further in later chapters. In addition, certain individuals are quite dramatically affected by the loss of light during the fall and winter months, developing a clinical syndrome known as *Seasonal Affective Disorder*, or *SAD*, which we'll discuss in the next section.

The Light/Depression Connection

For millions of people, the arrival of autumn signals not the pleasure associated with the scent of burning leaves or the refreshing crispness of the air. Instead they find themselves experiencing a darkening of the spirit. An estimated 15 percent of adult Americans suffer from SAD, and for them, the fall (and less often the spring or summer) is a harbinger of depression.

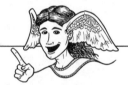

Morpheus Says

The relationship between SAD and the shorter period of daylight that occurs during the fall and winter months is even more pronounced in northern climates. According to the National Institute of Mental Health, about 9.7 percent of New Hampshire residents suffer from this disorder, whereas only 1.4 percent of Floridians do. This clearly points out the relationship between day lengths and SAD: Days become shorter and shorter the more northern the latitude.

People with SAD usually suffer from the same symptoms as other clinically depressed patients—feelings of sadness, helplessness, hopelessness, guilt, and mild illness. Unlike most of their counterparts, however, they tend to eat more rather than less during this time, experience weight gain, and crave rich carbohydrates. They spend many more hours than usual asleep, yet feel chronically exhausted and lethargic. Researchers now believe that the problem in people with SAD is that they are highly sensitive to the changes in day length that occur during the autumn and winter, and that their biological rhythms fall out of synch as a result.

Depression may result because the amount of sunlight to which we are exposed affects the production and use not only of the hormone melatonin (which is a sleep promoter), but also of the neurotransmitters serotonin and norepinephrine (which are intimately connected with mood). In 1997, a study published in *Nature* suggested that light therapy may ease depression by helping boost levels of serotonin. Those people who suffer from SAD benefit from receiving regular doses of bright light in the early morning, which tricks the brain into perceiving that the days are longer than they really are, and, in turn, this triggers the release of serotonin.

Switching It On...and Off

Whether you suffer from SAD or from another sleep problem, the best way for you to get all the bright light you need is to simply go outside into the sun, if you live in a climate with lots of it, or to use a light box or one of the other alternatives we describe later in the chapter.

If you're an Owl who wants to wake up a little earlier, for instance, you should try to get out into the early morning light for a few days and you may see a shift in your natural sleep/wake patterns. At the same time, it's important to plan your periods of darkness with care, too. The Lark who wants to shift his or her clock forward a bit, for instance, should remain in the dark in the early morning hours, even if awake.

Unfortunately, not everyone lives in a climate or has a work schedule that permits regular, well-timed exposure to the sun. People who live in regions with long, dark winters or excessively overcast climates may have more difficulty maintaining their natural sleep/wake cycle (they also run a greater risk of developing SAD). Other people who could benefit from the right light at the right time are those who work the night shift or travel across time zones and want to avoid exhaustion and jet lag.

Two sleep disorders called *Advanced Sleep Phase Syndrome (ASPS)* and *Delayed Sleep Phase Syndrome (DSPS)* are also related to the effects of light on the

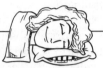

Sleep on it

The human body is especially sensitive to light at night: Even the relatively dim light provided by regular light bulbs can have a stimulating effect. If you have trouble getting to sleep at night, try turning off all but the most necessary lights in your home and even reading by a relatively dim light (75 watts or less) focused directly on the book or magazine you're reading.

Night Owl Wisdom

Advanced Sleep Phase Syndrome (ASPS) and Delayed Sleep Phase Syndrome (DSPS) are two sleep problems related to a disruption of the circadian clock. ASPS is more rare and involves the tendency to wake up very, very early in the morning—sometimes before 4 a.m. DSPS is more common and involves the inability to fall asleep until quite late, sometimes not before 2 or 3 a.m.

biological clock. People who suffer from ASPS become sleepy very early in the evening and wake up very early in the morning. When left to their own devices, those with Delayed Sleep Phase Disorder get up very late in the morning and cannot fall asleep until the wee hours just before dawn. On vacations or weekends, both groups sleep well, once they get to sleep, but do so out of synch with the rest of the world. The problem comes when they try to conform to normal business hours. A person with DSPS who must rise at 6 or 7 a.m. for work becomes severely sleep deprived when he or she cannot fall asleep until 3 or 4 a.m. Likewise, a person with ASPS who tries to conform to social pressure in the evening and stays awake until 10 or 11 p.m. gets similarly sleep deprived because he or she naturally wakes up at 2 or 3 a.m. Researchers believe that those who suffer from ASPS or DSPS may lack a sensitivity to light that would otherwise naturally reset their body clocks and keep them in synch.

Finding the Right Light

Unfortunately, even if you turned all the lights on in your house and stood naked beneath them, it would be difficult to receive enough artificial light to significantly shift your internal biological rhythms—unless you exposed yourself to light at precisely the same time each day. As mentioned earlier in this chapter, if you stand in a room lit with 75- or 100-watt light bulbs, you'll receive only about 200 to 500 lux, far less than what you receive from exposure to sunlight. And most studies show that light's effect on circadian rhythms is "dose dependent," meaning that the longer and brighter the exposure, the greater the effect on the timing of the biological clock.

The good news is that technology has come to the rescue once again. In recent years, several companies (and we list some of them in Appendix A) have developed light boxes and other products to provide bright, full-spectrum light in the home. Prices for these devices range from as little as $300 to as much as $1,000 (or more for larger systems). The most efficient ones have special high-intensity fluorescent tubes that use just 150 watts of electricity (and thus cost less than a penny a day to run).

Here are a few of the answers technology has provided:

➤ *Light boxes.* Light boxes typically measure about two feet by three feet and enclose a full-spectrum light or bright white light that you can angle toward your face. You can sit about 18 inches away and dose yourself with 5,000 to 10,000 lux of light by keeping your head and eyes turned toward the light—without looking directly into it while reading or doing other tasks. The time and length of your sessions would vary, depending on your purpose (for example, shifting your circadian rhythm or alleviating the winter blues).

➤ *Light visors.* Light visor models, which you wear like sun visors, are powered by rechargeable batteries. They usually offer about 2,500 lux brightness. Small lights fit under the visor and shine light directly above your eyes. Wearing one feels just like wearing a baseball cap, except your face is bathed in light.

➤ *Wall units.* These are often designed to look like a window that receives natural light, and frequently come complete with outdoor scene screens. They provide full-spectrum ambient light, so it's almost like being outside in the sun right in your living room. Unfortunately, although they may be more attractive, many of these devices do not produce the same light intensity as do the other systems.

Some light boxes include dusk/dawn lighting controls that simulate natural spring/ summer light cycles. You can also get one that you can program yourself so that you can simulate (or enhance) sunrise in the morning and darkness falling at night in your bedroom. This way it is possible to awaken from Stage 2 or REM sleep when one will feel most refreshed.

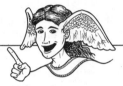

Morpheus Says

When it comes to treating SAD, the timing of exposure to bright light is directed at increasing the photo period (the virtual daylight length). According to a landmark paper by Alfred Lewy, M.D., published in *Psychiatric Annals* in 1987, people suffering from SAD are best served by exposure to 10,000 lux for 30 minutes or one to two hours of 2,500 lux exposure as soon as they wake up. However, if they experience the common depression-related symptom of early morning awakening, they should wait until 6 or 7 a.m. before they begin treatment.

Risks and Side Effects

The side effects of light therapy are minimal, if any. In the beginning of treatment, some people do react to the intense lights, sometimes with a feeling of unease or nausea. These symptoms tend to pass with time. Another common side effect is dry eyes, which you can easily alleviate by applying artificial tears (such as Visine) or by running a humidifier. Headaches, eyestrain, and irritability may also occur.

Although most light boxes do not emit dangerous ultraviolet rays that could permanently damage your eyes, it's best to avoid looking directly into the light source. At the very least, you're apt to strain your eyes, and you may even develop a mild

Wake Up!

DO NOT undergo light therapy if you have any eye problems such as retinitis pigmentosa, diabetic retinopathy, or macular degeneration, until you have checked with your ophthalmologist and receive his or her advice and supervision. Otherwise, you risk serious and permanent eye damage.

headache from the experience. To avoid these problems, allow the light to enter your eyes indirectly. Place the box slightly above you so that the light falls on you like the rays of the sun.

If you experience unpleasant side effects, you can try decreasing the length of exposure or sit a little farther away from the unit.

Although we're lucky to be able to compensate for the lack of daylight with bright light technology, nothing really beats getting out into the natural sunlight if you've got it available to you (those of you surviving through northern winters or living in the naturally foggy Pacific Northwest may need some extra help!). You'll see in the next chapter that a brisk, 5- or 10-minute walk in the sun and fresh air can help you avoid those dips in concentration and energy that so often occur to the sleep-deprived.

The Least You Need to Know

➤ Light is an important signal to our internal clocks.

➤ Without sufficient and well-timed exposure to bright light, your mood and your sleep/wake patterns may become disrupted.

➤ Light boxes and other devices, when used in your home or office, can mimic the bright light you'd receive from the sun.

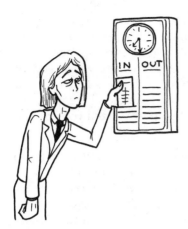

Chapter 12

Getting Through the Day

In This Chapter

➤ Exploring sleep deprivation and its effects

➤ The dangers of drowsy driving

➤ Tips for staying alert

According to a 1997 National Sleep Foundation/Gallup poll, more than 63 million Americans suffer dangerous levels of sleep deprivation, and nearly four in ten of those people reported that daytime sleepiness interferes with their day-to-day activities at least some of the time.

How about you? Did you take the Sleepiness Quotient Quiz in Chapter 5? How did you score? If you have any reason to believe that you're not getting enough sleep on a regular basis, and if you are attempting to function at optimal levels when your body is overtired, then read on. This chapter will help explain what happens when your body and brain go on the blink, and what you can do to prevent the worst from happening when they do. First, however, let's take a look at a subject you may have thought little about: What it really means to be alert.

The Meaning of Alertness

Back in Chapter 8, we discussed the "fight-or-flight response," the physiological event that occurs when the body and mind senses danger. As you may remember, your sympathetic nervous system becomes activated in emergency situations, which causes your heart to beat faster, your blood pressure to rise, your muscles to tense up, and your respiration rate to increase. When these physiological responses occur, your body

Night Owl Wisdom

The **parasympathetic nervous system** is the part of the autonomic nervous system responsible for relaxing or slowing down the body's activities after they have been stimulated by the sympathetic nervous system. The parasympathetic nervous system lowers blood pressure, decreases heart rate, and relaxes muscle fibers once a period of perceived emergency or hypervigilance passes.

is at its most alert and active: you're literally wide awake and ready for anything. But you have another part of your nervous system that takes over when the emergency has been resolved. The *parasympathetic nervous system* causes you to relax: It slows down your heart and respiration rates, lowers your blood pressure, and relaxes your muscles. And the more relaxed you are, the less alert you are.

When it comes to making it through a day (or night) when you're feeling sleepy, you'll want to do your best to "switch on" the sympathetic nervous system and "switch off" its counterpart, the parasympathetic nervous system. We'll show you how to do that later in the chapter. In the meantime, it's important to understand what can happen if you're not awake when you should be. Indeed, feeling sleepy when you're supposed to be awake, alert, and ready for action can be dangerous no matter what activity you're performing—except perhaps when you're sunbathing or watching afternoon soaps.

Measuring Alertness

How do you know when you're alert, when you're drowsy, or when you're about to fall asleep? And how do you know when your level of alertness is about to dip below the safety level? You might find those questions pretty hard to answer, and if so, you're not alone. Even laboratory tests designed to measure and evaluate alertness have trouble isolating the elements involved in these conditions.

Thanks to the widespread study of sleep with the use of the polysomnograph (the machine that measures brain waves and other signals), we have gained some understanding of what alertness is, and what happens when it's lost. The standard laboratory test used to assess alertness today is the Multiple Sleep Latency Test (MSLT). As described in Chapter 4, this test determines the time it takes a person to fall asleep in a darkened room. A person with a very low alertness level will drop off in less than five minutes or so, while an alert person will spend the entire allotted bed time of 20 minutes wide awake.

When combined with information about how much the subject slept the night before, the MSLT allows us to put numbers on the relative effects of the loss of sleep. The following figures show what happens to alertness depending on the number of hours of lost sleep and then what happens over time if you lose just two hours of sleep each night.

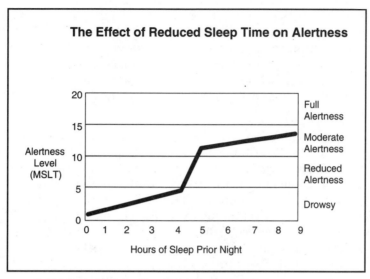

As you can see from this graph, the less sleep you receive at night, the less alert you are the following day. Notice that the difference between getting 5 hours and 9 hours sleep during a single night is relatively small, but if you get less than 5 hours of sleep (3 full sleep cycles), your alertness levels take a perilous dip the next day.

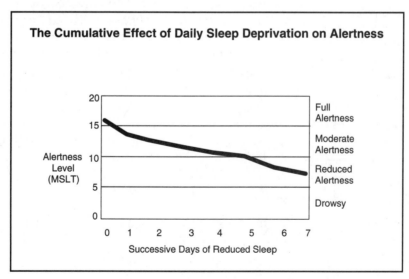

This graph shows the cumulative effects of a loss of just 2 hours of sleep every night over the course of a week. The first day after such a loss you might not fare so poorly, but by the fifth, sixth, or seventh day, your alertness level has fallen to a dangerous level.

141

Indeed, the loss of just a few hours of sleep can considerably reduce your level of alertness just when you may need it most. You've read some of the statistics about the high costs of sleep deprivation in Chapter 1, but it's important to reiterate some of them here. Did you know, for instance, that the primary cause of the Three Mile Island accident, in which a Pennsylvania nuclear power plant nearly experienced a core meltdown, occurred because of operator carelessness and inattention in the wee hours of the morning?

Without question, fatigued people make errors. And while most such errors are on a much smaller scale than the Three Mile Island disaster, taken together they have an enormous effect. Remember, when the body and brain fail to get the rest they need, certain functions become impaired. You can't concentrate as well, your reaction time is slower, your creative juices certainly aren't flowing, and your mood, well, that's just shot. Sometimes you merely get through your day on "automatic pilot." You simply go through the motions without really thinking about them. Unfortunately, this phenomenon, known as *automatic behavior*, is probably the real reason that so many accidents occur to sleep-deprived people. Examples of automatic behavior include a railroad engineer who can continue pressing a safety lever at regular intervals but doesn't notice an obstruction on the track, and a trucker who keeps his rig on the road but misses his intended exit.

Night Owl Wisdom

Automatic behavior refers to a period of several minutes when a sleep-deprived person is able to continue performing routine duties but is incapable of active cognition—which means he or she can carry out a task without thinking about what's really occurring at the time.

Microsleeps, which we first described in Chapter 1, are another dangerous side effect of sleep deprivation and night shift work. These brief, involuntary episodes of sleep may last only a few seconds, but they cause an interruption of thought and behavior that can result in serious mistakes at work or on the road.

While many accidents related to sleep deprivation occur at night—and we'll explore that problem further in Chapter 15—there's no question that sleep deprivation also takes a toll on those of us who work during the day. And nowhere is this more evident than on the nation's highways and byways.

Asleep at the Wheel

Before we discuss perhaps the most frightening consequence of sleep deprivation—drowsy driving—take this quiz to see how much you already know.

The Drowsy Driving Awareness Quiz

Answer these questions "True" or "False."

1. I can tell when I'm about ready to nod off.
   True _____   False _____

2. I'm a safe driver, so it doesn't matter if I'm sleepy.
   True _____   False _____

3. A cup of coffee is all I need to wipe out the effects of sleep deprivation and stay alert during a long drive.
   True _____   False _____

4. Young people need less sleep.
   True _____   False _____

Copyright © 1998 by Circadian Information Limited Partnership. Reprinted with permission. All rights reserved.

How many times did you answer "True"? The more often you did, the less you understand about the nature of drowsy driving. Let's see where you went wrong.

1. If you're really drowsy, you probably won't know when you're about to fall asleep. You also won't be able to tell how long you were "out" if you do nod off, and being asleep even for a few seconds can kill you or someone else.

2. The only safe driver is an alert driver. Consider this: The young man awarded the title of "America's Safest Driver" in 1990 later fell asleep at the wheel and was killed.

3. Food or drinks containing caffeine, such as chocolate, coffee, or cola, can help you feel alert—but only for a short time. If you drink coffee while seriously sleep deprived, you're still likely to suffer the brief 4- or 5-second naps called microsleeps. At 60 miles an hour, a five-second microsleep will leave you 150 yards down the road, and perhaps in the middle of a head-on collision.

4. Young people are no less immune to sleep deprivation than their older counterparts. In fact, teenagers and those in their 20s need relatively more sleep than people in their 40s and older—but they tend to get less because they like to stay up later than they should. That's why, in addition to teaching young people about the dangers of drunk driving, many experts recommend adding a segment on drowsy driving to standard Drivers' Education classes.

How'd you do? If you got even one or two answers wrong, you might just be putting yourself and others at risk by driving when your alertness levels are less than optimal. According to the U.S. National Highway Traffic Safety Administration, driver fatigue is the primary cause of at least 100,000 police-reported crashes and more than 1,500 deaths annually. And a 1995 National Sleep Foundation Gallup Survey found that 52 percent of adult Americans have driven while drowsy and 31 percent have, at some time, fallen asleep at the wheel.

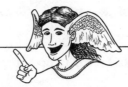

Morpheus Says

Professional truck drivers—faced with tight deadlines that force them to drive irregular, extended hours—are even more likely than regular travelers to become sleep deprived. Indeed, a study of American and Canadian long-haul truck drivers published in the September 11, 1997, *New England Journal of Medicine* found that a large percentage of these workers are getting fewer than five hours of sleep per night.

Drowsy driving is all too common, especially among young men aged 25 and under. Night-shift workers who rotate their schedules are also at high risk, a fact we'll discuss in more depth in Chapter 15. Others at risk include people who regularly drive long distances, such as truck drivers, and those who have insomnia or other sleep problems.

Here are some of the symptoms of drowsy driving:

➤ Your eyes go out of focus or close.

➤ You have trouble keeping your head up.

➤ You can't stop yawning.

➤ You have trouble concentrating.

➤ You realize you don't remember driving the last few miles.

➤ You drift between lanes, tailgate, or miss traffic signs.

➤ You drift off the road or narrowly miss crashing.

A little later in this chapter you'll learn some general tips about staying awake during the day. In the meantime, here are some tips specifically designed to help you drive safely at any hour:

➤ *Rest up.* Get enough sleep the night before, and plan to drive during times of the day when you normally feel most alert and awake.

➤ *Choose your time wisely.* Avoid driving during your body's "down times," which are, for Regular Robins, during the mid-afternoon and then

Just for You!

For all of you Owls out there, don't try to start a long drive early in the morning when you're least likely to feel alert. Instead, plan to begin later in the morning or in the early evening. Larks, on the other hand, do best driving in the early morning hours, then knocking off by evening.

between midnight and 6 a.m. (See the "Basic-Rest Activity Cycle—for Larks and Owls" figure in Chapter 13 to see what we mean.)

➤ *Drive with a buddy.* Not only can you share driving responsibilities, but you can also monitor each other's signs of drowsiness and help each other stay awake. When driving through the night, BOTH of you should stay awake. If your buddy goes to sleep while you're driving, there'd be no one left to monitor your level of alertness.

➤ *Take breaks.* Schedule a break every two hours or every 100 miles—but stop sooner if you show any danger signs of sleepiness. During your break, stretch, take a walk, and eat a light snack before getting back into the car. If you're sleepy, take a 10- or 20-minute nap.

Read on for more tips, some of which you can use to help you stay alert while driving.

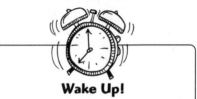

Wake Up!

For safety's sake, if you need to stop driving to catch a nap, do so only in a safe, well-lit, heavily-trafficked travel plaza or truck stop—and always lock your doors.

Easy Pick Ups

In the best of all possible worlds, you'd get all the sleep you need every night, work regular hours throughout your career, never have to care for an infant or parent in the middle of the night, and thus wake up every day feeling terrific.

But you're in the real world, aren't you? And so you have days when you're just not feeling your best after a night of restless sleep, days that nonetheless require you to be every bit as perky and efficient as you would be with a full night's sleep. On days like that, you need some help, don't you? Well, that's what we're here for. Here are some tips we hope will help you make the most of those kinds of days:

➤ *Rise to the challenge.* Performing a boring, routine task when you're already feeling drowsy just about puts you over the edge, doesn't it? But if you've got something new and preferably stimulating to do, you're apt to perk right up. In Chapter 15, we'll talk about how urgent such stimulation is when it comes to safety-sensitive jobs, such as those in the nuclear power industry. In the meantime, if you find yourself losing focus, switch to a more refreshing task until you feel better.

➤ *Move it or lose it.* Any type of muscular activity triggers the sympathetic nervous system and helps keep you alert—and you don't have to run a mile or lift weights for the activity to have a positive effect. Depending on how sleep deprived you are, a walk around the block or performing simple stretches at your desk may be enough to boost your alertness level for an hour or two. Even chewing gum can briefly give you a lift.

➤ *Cool off.* A blast of cool dry air helps raise your alertness level, especially if you've been lulled into drowsiness by sitting in a warm, humid environment. Open a window, run a fan, or—if you have this option—take a cool shower.

➤ *Aromatherapy 101.* Some researchers believe that aroma can play a role in enhancing alertness. For instance, a driving simulation study by the Institute for Circadian Physiology published in *Sleep Research* found that the scent of peppermint "had an alerting effect at the end of the night when the subjects were most sleepy." In this study, six volunteers drove during the overnight hours on two different nights. On one night, a peppermint scent was diffused into the driving simulation room every 10 minutes for 2 seconds. The drivers were exposed to unscented air the second night. The volunteers scored better on the night that they were exposed to the scent of peppermint.

A Healthy Diet Redux

Food can be your friend when you find yourself sleepy when you're supposed to be alert. In addition to following the healthy diet recommendations made back in Chapter 7, the following tips may help you through a rough, sleepy day:

➤ *Always eat breakfast.* If you don't eat breakfast, your body will be operating at an energy deficit when you need the fuel most.

➤ *Combine complex carbohydrates and protein.* A low-sugar, high-fiber cereal and low-fat milk or yogurt is a perfect meal for those just getting ready to go—the combination makes for long-lasting energy.

➤ *Avoid the high-sugar/high-carbohydrate rush.* Consuming sugar and carbohydrates like those found in doughnuts or pastries will trigger an energy rush at first, but then you'll crash. Carbohydrates, especially in combination with fat, trigger the release of serotonin, which will help calm you, but may also make you sleepy.

➤ *Monitor caffeine intake.* Although the first thing you reach for is a cup of coffee or tea when you're feeling sleepy, consuming too much caffeine can cause wild rises and dips in energy and mood, especially if you do so continuously on a daily basis. Limit your intake to one or two cups in the morning and one or two during your afternoon slump if you feel the need.

Prevention Is the Best Medicine

Clearly, a much easier way to win the battle against sleep deprivation is getting enough sleep to begin with. Since that's not always possible in one shot during the night, you may need to learn the fine art of napping. By using the nap to recover from a sleep loss or to give you an added boost in anticipation of a long night, you can avoid becoming another victim of sleep deprivation. Read Chapter 13 and see for yourself.

The Least You Need to Know

➤ Sleep deprivation is hazardous to your health—and the health of others!

➤ You can avoid an accident due to driving drowsy by being aware of the symptoms of drowsiness and getting yourself off the road before you put yourself and others in danger.

➤ Taking a walk, exposing yourself to bright light, and monitoring your intake of caffeine can help you stay alert when you feel sleepy.

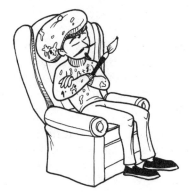

Chapter 13

The Art of the Nap

In This Chapter

➤ Napping as a biological function

➤ Napping as a cultural "ideal"

➤ Understanding your napping personality

➤ Tips for healthy napping—at home and at work

Cats and babies: For many people, these are the only creatures who do (or should) nap on a regular basis.

But nothing could be further from the truth. Built into the human circadian hardware are two major opportunities for sleep: One in the middle of the night and the other in mid-afternoon. For many people, taking a nap either on a regular basis or in order to make up for a sleep debt helps them function well throughout the day and, indeed, sleep better at night.

What about you? What did you find out about your napping nature back in Chapter 5? Can you—and do you—easily nap to make up for a sleep loss or to prepare for a particularly long night or day ahead? Or do you think napping is simply not part of your nature? (If you're really nap-o-phobic, you probably think napping is a waste of time no matter who's doing the napping!)

The fact is, if you really aren't getting the sleep that you need at night, you probably *can* learn to nap efficiently. In this chapter, we'll explore the nature of napping and then show you how to build a nap into your day. Then, in Chapters 17 and 18, we'll show you how napping can help you adjust more quickly to night-shift work and jet lag—two increasingly common activities that disrupt circadian rhythms.

The Culture of Napping

The human habit of consolidating sleep into one large, continuous block of 7 or 8 hours is fairly uncommon in the animal kingdom: Most animals, feline or not, "catnap," spreading out their sleep periods and activity periods throughout the day and night. Others (many of those in the rodent family, for instance) choose to sleep mostly during the day and stay awake—and hunt—during the night.

As you may remember from Chapter 1, anthropologists and biological historians remain unsure of why humans developed this nighttime sleep pattern, but one theory is that sleeping during the night kept us out of harm's way in the dark. Another possibility is that we need extended periods of unconsciousness in order to create, to build, to imagine…in short, to be human—and nighttime provides us with the best conditions under which to do so.

At the same time, however, the practice of napping—of sleeping during the day, imagine that!—has developed in many cultures around the world. You've no doubt heard of the "siesta"—the lovely Mediterranean and Latin American tradition of taking a post-lunch afternoon nap. In Mexico, for example, about 80 percent of adults indulge in an almost daily 90-minute nap. The siesta may have developed, at least in part, to give workers a rest during the hottest part of the afternoon, as well as to provide them with enough energy to work later into the evening hours.

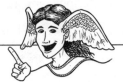

Morpheus Says

Dr. Gary Zammit, in his book *Good Nights* (Andrews and McMeel, 1997), points out that at least two communities—the Temiar people of Indonesia and the Iban of Sarawak—sleep about four hours a night and then nap many times during the day. This sleep pattern is termed "polyphasic," which simply means that sleep is achieved in several installments, so to speak, rather than in a single block of time during the night.

According to the 1997 National Sleep Foundation/Gallup Poll "Sleepiness in America," only about one in five Americans report that they take regular naps. Indeed, there remains a resistance to napping in our culture, even though sleep deprivation has become a major problem throughout the nation. In fact, although *planned napping* is apparently anathema to American go-getters, *unplanned napping*—while driving, while working, while at school—seems to be on the rise, leading to the loss of life as well as millions of dollars in lost productivity.

Fortunately, more and more companies are beginning to see the advantages of allowing—even encouraging—planned napping in the workplace. Especially helpful for night-shift and split-shift workers in 24-hour companies, napping as a strategy for increasing productivity is also showing up in industries that demand a high level of creativity, including advertising agencies, software development companies, and investment houses. Because judicious napping refreshes the creative mind and helps relieve stress, workers who "indulge" at the right time can then put in longer hours before losing motivation and inspiration.

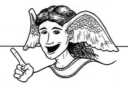

Morpheus Says

More and more companies are offering employees the chance to freshen up with a nap during work hours. For example, Circadian Technologies has helped the Burlington Northern & Santa Fe Railway Company develop a napping program for its train operators. So far, the company has applied a napping policy to about 10,000 workers and plans to extend the benefit to the remainder of its 43,000 employees.

Nevertheless, we've got a long way to go before most Americans consider napping a worthy enterprise and a habit worth cultivating. The signs are good, however, that the tide is turning. Napping rooms devoid of phones, faxes, or computer screens and equipped with cots or napping chairs are popping up in more and more workplaces every day.

Dispelling Napping Myths

Our resistance to napping here in the United States appears to be as much a part of our own culture as the siesta is in other societies. In fact, our "work through anything" mentality has spawned a few myths about napping that deserve to be dispelled here and now. These myths include:

➤ *To want to nap is an inherent sign of laziness.* First of all, you already know that you have a built-in, physiological desire for a nap in the mid-afternoon. While some people hardly feel that urge, or can suppress it quite easily, those of us who accept it (even relish it) are no less healthy or motivated. Second of all, just plain, good old-fashioned laziness (on your own time, of course) isn't such a bad thing on an occasional basis. Indeed, there's no rule that says you always have to be on the go throughout the daylight hours.

➤ *If you nap during the day, you won't sleep well at night.* This is one of the oldest myths about napping around. The truth is, napping during the day—if you're sleep deprived—can actually help you sleep *better* at night! Consider this: After having had a poor night's sleep and a long, busy day, have you ever then simply felt too anxious and stressed to sleep when you finally get to bed at night? That feeling can make it impossible for you to fall asleep and stay asleep. If you'd had a nap earlier that day, on the other hand, your body and mind would be under less stress and far more able to relax and sleep at night.

➤ *Mid-afternoon is the only time you're supposed to nap.* While the mid-afternoon (around 2 or 3 p.m.) is when most people find it easiest to nap, no specific time is completely off-limits. Remember, we each have our own unique internal clocks that help to set our daily rhythms. Remember Oliver the Owl, whom you met in Chapter 6? The times he would prefer to nap are very different from his Lark counterpart, Letitia. And a Regular Robin may have a much more flexible napping ability than his Owl and Lark counterparts. If you listen to your own body and take advantage of its natural lulls and dips, you'll be able to find the most comfortable and successful time to nap for you. Avoid napping within a few hours of your bedtime, however, which can keep you up at night.

➤ *Long naps are better than short naps.* Although it may seem unlikely, the truth is that a 15- to 30-minute nap can be just as refreshing in certain situations as a longer nap of 90 to 100 minutes—and it will clearly be superior to one that lasts from 45 minutes to an hour. That's because of the architecture of sleep (described in Chapter 3)—at 45 minutes, you are half-way through the 90-minute sleep cycle and in the deepest stages of sleep. Indeed, carefully timing a nap to make it either very short or long can make all the difference in the world.

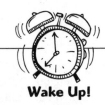

Wake Up!

Monitor the effects of naps on your nighttime sleep with care. If you find it hard to sleep at night but nap nearly every day, you may want to cut down on, or cut out, your daytime naps. Remember, you only need to sleep a certain number of hours each day to feel rested and alert. Too long a nap at the wrong time (especially within a few hours of bedtime) is bound to affect the quality of your major sleep period at night.

The 90-Minute Sleep Cycle

Drowsiness, then deeper and deeper sleep, then a state of active but unconscious brain activity, then almost awake again, and then back down into deep sleep—so goes the sleep cycle, which takes about 90 to 100 minutes. We travel through this remarkable cycle several times a night.

What you might not realize is that the 90-minute sleep cycle is part of a larger pattern of rest and activity that continues throughout the day. Known as the *basic rest-activity cycle*, or BRAC, this pattern explains why there are times when you feel especially alert and times when you're desperate for a cup of caffeine or a burst of fresh air to stimulate you. These "down times" represent the times when the circuits complete more slowly, when the vestiges of a catnapping ancestry show through. The BRAC cycles are usually very subtle, and we are usually able to either ignore them or to compensate for them with caffeine or other forms of stimulation. (It's no accident that the typical workplace coffee break takes place at 10:30, 90 minutes after work begins and, for many people, 180 minutes after getting out of bed at 7:30.)

Although the BRAC pattern is most pronounced at night when you'd normally be in bed asleep, you also experience it during the day. Becoming aware of your daily fluctuations up and down the alertness wave (see the following figure) will help you find the best naptime for your body and mind. In fact, there are two reasons to understand the 90-minute rhythm: First, you'll be able to better choose a time when you're more likely to fall asleep. Second, you'll know about how long to sleep in order to wake up feeling refreshed and ready to go instead of groggy and out-of-sorts.

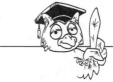

Night Owl Wisdom

The **basic rest-activity cycle (BRAC)** is the 90- to 100-minute oscillation of brain waves signaling the rise and fall of alertness that continues throughout the day and night.

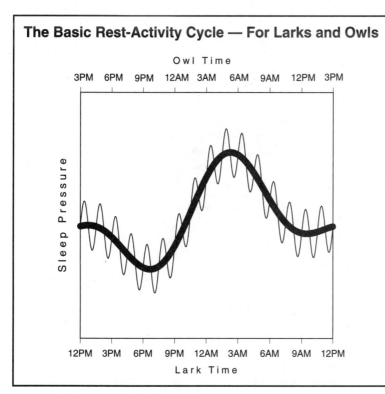

The Basic Rest-Activity Cycle — For Larks and Owls

Owl Time

3PM 6PM 9PM 12AM 3AM 6AM 9AM 12PM 3PM

Sleep Pressure

12PM 3PM 6PM 9PM 12AM 3AM 6AM 9AM 12PM

Lark Time

This graph shows both the 90-minute BRAC (the lighter lines) and the daily (dark line) dips and rises in sleep pressure. In Owl Time, the greatest pressure to sleep starts building at about midnight, while for Larks, it starts about 3 hours earlier, at 9 p.m. Following the BRAC line, you can see that there are times during the day when your sleep pressure is greater, and thus the opportunity for napping more pronounced.

The best time to start to nap during any 90-minute cycle is at the point when you first start to feel drowsy...not when you're already having trouble keeping your eyes open. If you get into napping position and close your eyes at that time, your body and mind can take full advantage of the 10- or 20-minute down-swing of alertness during that cycle. If you can afford it and are particularly sleep-deprived, you could sleep for a whole 90 minutes, going through all four stages of sleep plus a whole REM (dreaming cycle).

However—and this is a big however—if you can't make it through a whole sleep cycle, you'll want to limit your nap to just 10 to 30 minutes. That way, you won't interrupt the deepest stages of REM sleep, which can leave you feeling worse than when you started. In fact, there's a strange thing that happens when you're awakened from a deep sleep called *sleep inertia*. Your arms and legs feel paralyzed, your vision is blurry, and you have difficulty concentrating. Sleep inertia usually lasts only about 30 minutes or so, but some people who wake up like this feel off-kilter for the rest of the day. Timing your sleep period so that you don't wake up during a REM cycle is the best way to avoid sleep inertia.

Although it may seem complicated at first, with a little practice you can learn to nap when your body and mind most crave a break, and then wake up feeling refreshed and ready to go. By timing your naps this way you'll help yourself avoid the dangers and the discomfort of sleep inertia.

Night Owl Wisdom

Sleep inertia is the term used to describe a set of symptoms usually related to waking up from the deep stages of sleep.

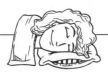

Sleep on it

If you know you're going to have a very late night—or even pull an all-nighter for one reason or another—you can take a "prophylactic" nap during the afternoon. Studies show that taking a 90-minute nap before staying awake all night increases alertness and performance by about 30 percent.

Making It Work for You

Winston Churchill went all the way, stripping down to his skivvies and climbing into bed for a nap that lasted a good hour and a half. Other nappers simply lean back in their chairs, close their eyes, and drift off to sleep for just 10 or 15 minutes.

How, when, and, indeed, *if* you nap depends on your Nap-Ability, as well as other aspects of your Sleep Personality, as assessed in Chapter 5. Take another look at how you scored, then read on to find out how best to incorporate naps into your life.

Who Naps When?

Generally speaking, the best time to doze is mid-afternoon. That's when our alertness levels are normally at their lowest and, if we're running a little short of sleep, it's easiest and most refreshing to nap at that time.

But that's just a general rule. As you learned in Chapter 5, each of us has a special Sleep Personality that helps determine if, when, and how we nap:

➤ *Long Sleepers.* Obtaining nine or ten uninterrupted hours of sleep—what long sleepers crave and require—is often impossible, especially for working parents or people who want to have an evening social life but who have to get up early in the morning for work. For long sleepers short on available night time, an afternoon or early-evening nap can make up the difference and keep them feeling alert and refreshed.

➤ *Short Sleepers.* Those of you who consistently get less than six hours of sleep per night could probably use the boost you get from grabbing a bit of shut-eye at some point during the day—and you probably could use that boost on a regular basis. However, if you feel awake and alert throughout the day, you shouldn't feel *obligated* to nap just because you naturally sleep less than the "norm" of 7 hours. Again, let your natural rhythms and needs help you determine a sleep/wake, rest/activity schedule that works for you.

➤ *Split Sleepers.* There are people out there who quite naturally (or at least easily) divide their wake periods into two portions, pretty much on a daily basis. They may sleep 4 to 6 hours during the night then, about 8 hours later, sleep another 1 to 3 hours. In essence, split sleepers live two "mini" days in the course of a single regular one and enjoy a restful, rejuvenating sleep period in-between each of their 8-hour days. As you can imagine, split sleepers are perfect night workers, and can easily adapt to time-zone changes.

➤ *Rigid Larks.* Remember Letitia the Lark, who simply couldn't sleep later in the morning no matter what time she got to bed at night? For Rigid Larks like her, taking a nap to either make up for a loss of sleep or prepare the body for a later-than-usual night is an essential strategy to avoid sleep deprivation.

➤ *Night Owls.* Oliver the Owl and his late-night brethren, on the other hand, make up for losses they suffer when having to get up earlier than usual by taking short naps in the evening. Oliver takes a 20-minute nap around 8 p.m., which refreshes him enough to make it through to his usual bedtime of about midnight. If he goes to bed for the night when he's exhausted at 8 or 9 p.m., on the other hand, he's liable to sleep until 1 a.m. and then be up all night.

➤ *Regular Robins.* Some Regular Robins (those people who have relatively "normal" sleep schedules that start between about 11 and midnight and finish at 6:30 or 7:30 a.m.) stay "regular" by taking a nap whenever they feel sleep deprived. They aren't split sleepers,

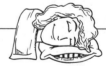

Sleep on it

Napping can be your best strategy for coping with the change that comes from Daylight Savings Time. After you turn your clocks forward on that springtime Sunday morning, get up at your regular time according to the clock that day. Make up for the loss with a nap in the afternoon, then go to bed at your normal time.

however, so naps are rarely a regular part of their routine. In most cases, Regular Robins are best able to nap in the mid-afternoon.

Tips for Healthy Napping

No matter who you are or when you nap, it's just as important to practice good sleep hygiene during these shorter sleep periods as it is at night. Here are some tips to help you become a better napper:

➤ *Stick to a routine.* As much as possible, get your body "in the mood" for a nap by following a pre-nap routine. If it's a short nap you're aiming for, performing a few simple stretches and loosening your tie or collar might be enough. If you're going for a long nap, you might want to follow (as much as possible) the same pre-bed routine you do at night—brushing your teeth, reading for a few minutes, and so on. This routine can even work at the office, as long as it doesn't involve changing into your pj's and clutching your teddy bear.

➤ *Batten down the hatches.* Even if you're taking a short 10- or 20-minute nap, take a few minutes (starting as soon as you feel drowsy) to turn off the lights, unplug the phone, and get as comfortable as possible. If you're taking a 90-minute nap, it's especially important to free your environment of all distractions.

➤ *Take advantage of your napping "windows of opportunity."* Once you start to feel drowsy, you're on the down-swing of a BRAC (basic rest-activity cycle). At that point, your body is ready to nap. If you try to nap when you're feeling alert, on the other hand, chances are you simply won't be able to, no matter how sleep-deprived you are.

➤ *Go short or long.* Again, you want to avoid that middle ground—the 40- or 50-minute nap that interrupts your deepest stages of sleep or your REM cycle. Otherwise you risk waking up feeling groggy and out-of-sorts—just the symptoms you wanted to avoid by taking a nap. Unless you can go for the whole 90 minutes, set an alarm clock to wake you after 10 or 20 minutes.

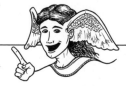

Morpheus Says

If you've got access to the Internet, you can join the World Nap Organization, a self-proclaimed "Open Society for the Advancement and Study of Napping." According to its Web page, its purpose involves:

➤ Proclaiming that we are nap takers

➤ Disregarding the disapproval of opponents of napping

➤ Educating ourselves and others about the positive effects of napping

➤ Collaborating on original research in napping

For more information, visit their Web site at www.bluemarble.net/~amyloo/wno.html.

And there you have it: Napping strategies for every Sleep Personality—and that includes yours. As you head into the 21st century along with the rest of us, it's likely that the demands on your time will become even greater and more pressing. It's essential—for your health and sanity—to keep your body and mind as rested and refreshed as possible. Indeed, napping may be the "wonder drug" of the new millennium!

The Least You Need to Know

➤ Napping is a natural part of the human circadian cycle.

➤ Take advantage of the several napping "windows of opportunity" you have throughout the day.

➤ Choosing when and how long to nap can mean the difference between waking up refreshed and feeling worse off than when you started.

➤ Maintaining proper sleep hygiene is as important for napping during the day as it is for sleeping at night.

Part 3
Under Special Circumstances

Do you snore? Walk in your sleep? Wake up in terror? Wake up way too early or stay up way too late? Or do you know someone with one or more of these sleep problems? We bet there are quite a few of you out there because clinical sleep disorders are far more common than you may think. The trouble is, if you don't treat your sleep disorder, a good night's sleep will remain as elusive as ever, no matter how good your sleep hygiene becomes. And you'll still have trouble sleeping if you're a frequent traveler who isn't able to manage jet lag or a night shift worker who hasn't learned the ins and outs of timing your sleep well so that you can work and live in health and with vitality.

But don't despair. Part 3 will help explain such special circumstances and provide you with plenty of tips to alleviate your particular problem.

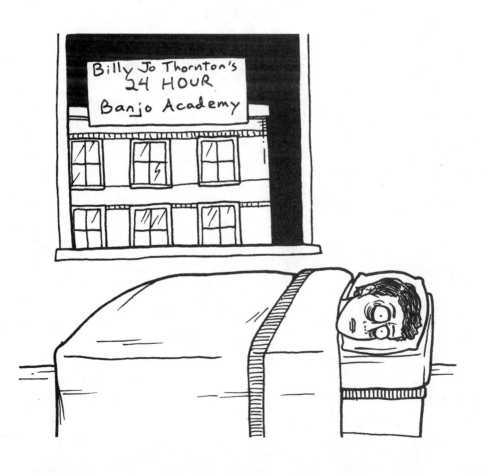

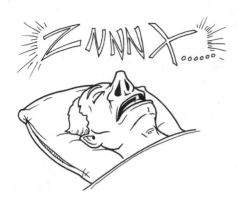

Chapter 14

The Big Snore

In This Chapter

➤ Understanding snoring and sleep apnea

➤ Defining the risks and side effects of sleep apnea

➤ Exploring some solutions to snoring and sleep apnea

"Laugh and the world laughs with you. Snore, and you sleep alone." So goes perhaps the most famous and eloquent observation, made by author Anthony Burgess, about this very common—and very disruptive—sleep problem. A potent destroyer of the marriage bed and the subject of endless jokes and comedy bits, snoring can be either a mild annoyance or a sign of a serious health condition. In fact, snoring and its close relative, Obstructive Sleep Apnea, represent the most common sleep problems in the United States.

In this chapter, we'll help all of you snorers—and your partners—gain some insight into the problem, determine its severity, and offer some potential solutions.

Snoring Is NOT FUNNY

Ranging from the gentle rumble of an undercurrent to a raging, snorting cacophony, the sounds of snoring disturb millions of households every night. (And snoring can be dangerous to your health in more ways than one: Legend has it that infamous Texas gunfighter John Wesley Hardin killed a snorer who disturbed his sleep by shooting him through the wall of his adjoining hotel room.) Today, snoring is extremely common. About 25 percent of all men snore each night; about half as many women snore. Unusual among young people, the prevalence of snoring increases after the age of 35.

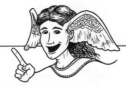

Morpheus Says

According to the *Encyclopedia of Sleep and Dreaming*, the word *snore* derives from the 11th- to 15th-century low German (*snorren*), Dutch (*snarren*), and English (*snoren*) words meaning "to drone" or "to hum." Although we tend to use "snore" to describe the noise made during sleep, the word also refers to the noise a ship makes when it cuts the waves with a roar.

Plainly speaking, snoring is a noise produced when an individual breathes during sleep (usually when the sleeper breathes *in*). This, in turn, causes the soft palate and *uvula* (you know, that thing that hangs down in the back of your throat) to vibrate. Sometimes, vibrations of the tongue, tonsils, and sides of the throat also contribute to the sound of snoring.

In addition to so-called "simple snoring," there is a medical condition—a potentially quite serious one—called Obstructive Sleep Apnea. With sleep apnea, a sleep disorder suffered by about 2 to 4 percent of middle-aged adults, the upper airway becomes completely obstructed for 10 seconds or longer, and often many times—sometimes hundreds of times—during the night. Although it's a serious medical disorder, more than 80 percent of sleep apneics fail to understand the problem or get medical help for it. And that's unfortunate because successful treatment can mean significant relief.

Night Owl Wisdom

The **uvula** is the small, soft extension of the soft palate that hangs from the roof of the mouth above the root of the tongue. It is composed of muscle, connective tissue, and mucous membrane.

The relationship between snoring and sleep apnea is a close one. By definition, all sleep apneics snore. Furthermore, recent research suggests that, over time, simple snoring can damage the tissues in the throat and nasal passages, making the development of sleep apnea more likely. As we'll discuss in this chapter, both snoring and sleep apnea can have serious health consequences and should never be taken lightly.

What Goes Wrong

Although most bed partners believe that snoring is simply a dastardly plot to keep them awake in the most annoying way possible, people who snore are anatomically different than their non-snoring counterparts. Among the differences that help create the problem—differences that are more pronounced in Obstructive Sleep Apnea than in simple snoring—are:

➤ *Poor muscle tone in the muscles of the tongue and throat.* This condition allows the tongue to fall backwards into the airway or the sides of the throat to close together.

➤ *Excessive bulkiness of the throat.* Being overweight and having a large neck size often contribute to snoring. Large tonsils and adenoids also commonly cause snoring in children.

➤ *Excessive length of the soft palate and uvula.* A long palate may narrow the opening from the nose into the throat. As it dangles in the airway, it acts as a flutter valve during relaxed breathing and contributes to the noise of snoring. A long uvula may make matters even worse.

➤ *Obstructed nasal airways.* When you have a stuffy or blocked-up nose, you have to inhale even harder to get enough air into your lungs. This creates an exaggerated vacuum in the throat—the collapsible part of the airway—that pulls together the floppy tissues of the throat. This phenomenon explains why some people snore only during hay fever season or when they have a cold or sinus infection.

In most cases, snoring is fairly simple and straightforward. It isn't horribly loud or raucous and it doesn't wake you up or disturb your sleep. Now, that doesn't mean that even simple snoring can't be serious: If it bothers your bed partner, it's serious. You may slumber the night away and wake up feeling refreshed, while your bedmate tosses and turns for hours and suffers from sleep deprivation the next day.

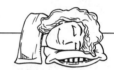

Sleep on it

If your partner's snoring keeps you awake at night, you MUST take action in order to avoid chronic sleep deprivation yourself. In addition to showing him or her this chapter, you can buy earplugs or sleep in another room until your partner finds a solution to the snoring problem.

Is It Apnea?

This quiz will help you decide if your snoring is a mere annoyance or a potential health hazard. Again, please note that some recent research suggests that simple snoring may eventually lead to sleep apnea in some people.

Is it Snoring or Sleep Apnea?

1. Does your snoring disturb your bed partner?
   Never _____ Sometimes _____ Usually _____

2. Do you snore in all sleeping positions?
   Never _____ Sometimes _____ Usually _____

3. Do you ever wake suddenly because of snoring?
   Never _____ Sometimes _____ Usually _____

4. Are you tired when you have to get up in the morning?

Never ____ Sometimes ____ Usually ____

5. Are you tired during the day?
   Never ____ Sometimes ____ Usually ____

6. Do you fall asleep while at the movies, watching TV, or while listening to a lecture?
   Never ____ Sometimes ____ Usually ____

7. Do you stop breathing for several seconds between snores (you'll probably have to ask a bed partner for the answer to this question!)?
   Never ____ Sometimes ____ Usually ____

Night Owl Wisdom

Obstructive Sleep Apnea is a condition in which breathing temporarily stops during sleep because the tongue and other tissues block the back of the throat.

Wake Up!

You may not be aware that you suffer from Obstructive Sleep Apnea. The condition may cause only mild disturbances in your sleep—disrupting your normal cycle but not causing you to wake up and open your eyes. In fact, you may be completely unaware that you even *have* a problem.

Score yourself 1 point for every "Never," 2 points for every "Sometimes," and 3 points for every "Usually." If you scored between 7 and 10 points, your snoring falls into the mild annoyance category. If you scored between 11 and 15, your snoring is probably disturbing you and your bed partner and may require treatment. A score between 16 and 21 means that your snoring is significantly disrupting your sleep and may be putting you at risk for more serious problems.

A Break in Breathing

Sleep apnea is more than just loud snoring. If you suffer from this medical condition, you literally stop breathing while asleep. In most cases, a condition called *Obstructive Sleep Apnea* is the problem. What happens is that your tongue or other soft tissues fall back and either completely collapse or partially obstruct the airway. Oxygen levels drop, and your throat muscles contract as you struggle to breathe. This break can last from a few seconds up to a minute or even longer. Finally, your throat opens, and you gasp or let out a snort as air rushes in. You can then fall back asleep.

Those with severe cases of sleep apnea repeat this process dozens of times each hour, up to 500 or more times a night. If you suffer from sleep apnea, snorting and snoring may become such a part of the nightly routine that you have no memory of your spasmodic breathing or its effect on your sleep.

In addition to Obstructive Sleep Apnea, two other forms

of the condition exist:

➤ *Central Sleep Apnea.* This fairly rare condition affects mostly adults over the age of 60. The brain "forgets" to tell the breathing muscles to move, and thus the sleeper stops breathing for several seconds until he or she wakes up and starts breathing again.

➤ *Mixed Sleep Apnea.* This condition involves brief periods of Central Sleep Apnea followed by longer periods of Obstructive Sleep Apnea.

The Symptoms of Sleep Apnea

Again, sleep apnea is more than just loud or constant snoring. It is related to a host of often serious medical conditions. The risks associated with sleep apnea include:

➤ *Excessive daytime sleepiness.* Because their breathing problems cause them to wake up several times a night, sleep apneics suffer terribly from sleep deprivation. In addition to physical, social, and psychological discomfort, such sleepiness can result in serious traffic and on-the-job accidents.

➤ *Irregular heartbeat.* With each episode of apnea, the heart rate falls, then increases again at the termination of apnea. In a small number of cases (about 3 percent), a serious arrhythmia (irregular heart rhythm) develops.

➤ *High blood pressure.* Several studies show an increased risk of high blood pressure in people with sleep apnea, and they are more frequently diagnosed with high blood pressure than their healthy counterparts.

➤ *Heart disease and stroke.* Sleep apnea has been associated with an increased incidence of heart attacks and stroke. Sleep lab evaluations of male stroke patients show that 75 percent of them have significantly increased apneic events.

The relationship between cardiovascular disease (including high blood pressure, heart disease, and stroke) and sleep apnea is currently under investigation by the National Heart, Lung, and Blood Institute. The Institute is conducting a Sleep Heart Health Study in which the sleep patterns and habits of 6,000 Americans, 40 years and older, will be examined to see what, if any, connection exists between sleep apnea and cardiovascular disease. The study, which began in 1995, will be completed in 1999.

Despite these severe related conditions, the symptoms of sleep apnea may be vague and subtle. You may feel tired and sleepy during the day, even after what you perceive to be a full night's sleep. You may have a headache, feel irritable, and experience memory difficulties and problems with concentration. Depression, impotence or loss of sex drive, and anxiety are also common side effects.

Risk Factors for Obstructive Sleep Apnea

Obstructive Sleep Apnea is most common in middle age and more likely to strike men than women. One big risk factor appears to be body fat. Sixty percent of people with sleep apnea are overweight. Specifically, however, it is not the excess poundage, but the neck size that counts. Men with a neck circumference of 17 inches or larger (16 inches for women) are more likely to have their airway collapse while they sleep. So are people with double chins or with a lot of fat at the waist. Apnea usually worsens with age because the tissues in the throat become floppier and people tend to gain weight at this time. Men are more susceptible because they often have beefier throat tissues and are more likely to gather fat in their abdomen, neck, and shoulders than women—all factors that contribute to creating a narrower airway.

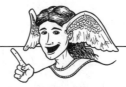

Morpheus Says

A study performed at the Osler Chest Unit of Churchill Hospital in Oxford, England, found that the only two factors that correlated with sleep apnea among 900 men were alcohol intake and neck size. The more alcohol the men consumed, the worse their symptoms, and the larger their neck size, the more likely they were to suffer from apnea.

There may be a genetic link as well. Snoring does run in families, and relatives of those affected with apnea tend to be more likely to have apnea and shallow breathing.

Diagnosing and Treating Sleep Apnea

If you think you may suffer from sleep apnea, talk to your doctor. He or she may suggest that you spend a night in a sleep laboratory to undergo special testing. Along with monitoring the stages of sleep you pass through and how long they last, the lab staff will measure your blood oxygen saturation, or the amount of oxygen your blood is carrying through your body, which indicates how much oxygen you inhale during sleep. They'll use an *oximeter*, which transmits a beam of light through a finger, toe, or ear and measures the wavelength of light that passes through. This measurement indicates the percentage of oxygen in the blood. Generally speaking, the less oxygen in the blood, the more severe your sleep apnea is likely to be: It means that you're not breathing in enough oxygen while you sleep.

Night Owl Wisdom

An **oximeter** is a device used to measure blood oxygen levels, an important diagnostic indicator of sleep apnea. The less oxygen in your blood, the more severely apnea is affecting your ability to breathe.

Once you know that you have sleep apnea and doctors have determined its severity, you can decide on the most appropriate treatment. Currently, the most effective treatment for moderate to severe sleep apnea is the CPAP, or Continuous Positive Airway Pressure. This device works during sleep by blowing air from a machine into a mask that you place over your nose. The air pressure keeps your airway open, thus eliminating the apnea and frequent awakenings. Once you can breathe normally during the night, you'll start to feel better almost immediately. Indeed, symptoms of daytime alertness often significantly improve after just one night and be completely back to normal in a week or two. Unfortunately, you have to continue to use CPAP throughout your life, unless you can lose sufficient weight or are one of the limited number of people who benefit from surgery.

These remarkable results tend to make up for the major drawback of CPAP, namely the mild discomfort the device causes at first. Most people get used to this setup quickly, however, especially when they realize how much better they feel during the day.

In some cases, your doctor may recommend surgery to treat your severe snoring and apnea. One technique, called the *uvuloplatopharyngoplasy*, or UPPP, reduces the size of the uvula, soft palate, or both. Only 50 percent of apneics have success with this technique. It is expensive and involves a painful recovery period. The newest surgical procedure zaps away excess tissue with a laser. Called a laser-assisted *uvulopalatoplasty* or LAUP, this procedure is less costly and requires a shorter and less painful recovery period than UPPP. On the downside, it often requires several treatments before it's effective.

Night Owl Wisdom

A **uvuloplatopharyngoplasy** is a surgical procedure that's used to reduce the size of the uvula, soft palate, or both. A **uvulopalatoplasty** is a laser surgery technique used to remove excess tissue from the back of the throat to reduce snoring and apnea.

You Don't Have to Sleep Alone

Snoring is not the easiest condition to cure, as the sheer number of devices and techniques developed to do so indicate. Indeed, more than 300 devices are registered in the U.S. Patent and Trademark Office as cures for snoring. Some are variations on the old idea of sewing a tennis ball on the pajama back to force the sleeper to avoid a back sleeping position, which tends to exacerbate snoring (see the following tip). Chin and head straps, neck collars, and devices inserted into the mouth are other options, though these may prove ineffective for your particular case. Many electrical devices have been designed to produce painful or unpleasant stimuli when snoring occurs. Again, the success rate is not remarkable, but some people do find that one or more of these gadgets can help.

Here are some healthful options for you to try (such as losing weight and cutting down on alcohol and caffeine) and others that may or may not help your particular situation.

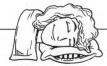

Sleep on it

To avoid rolling over on your back during the night, try stuffing a tennis ball into a sock and clip it to the back of your nightshirt.

➤ *Lose weight if you need to.* Even a relatively small loss in weight—say, 10 to 15 pounds—can make a difference when it comes to snoring and obstructive sleep apnea.

➤ *Change position.* Most snorers tend to sleep on their backs. If you do, try sleeping on your side or stomach to see if that makes a difference.

➤ *Avoid alcohol and tranquilizers.* These substances relax throat muscle tissue and depress breathing, thus making both snoring and apnea more likely.

➤ *Stop smoking.* Cigarette smoke can swell throat tissues, increase mucus formation, and worsen the low oxygen levels that accompany apnea.

➤ *Clear up stuffiness.* If you have a cold or suffer from allergies, use a decongestant that helps clear your nasal passages and makes it easier for you to breathe.

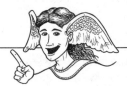

Morpheus Says

English bulldogs—you know, those "so ugly they're cute" sleepy pets with the pushed-in faces—also suffer from sleep apnea. Short-snouted bulldogs share many features with their human apneic counterparts: They have distorted nasal passages, a big tongue in a short jaw, and thick extra tissues around the throat near the opening of the windpipe.

➤ *Use a dental appliance.* A dentist can fit you with an oral device that repositions your tongue and jaw to hold them forward. Because it keeps the tongue from closing against the back of the throat, you may find such a device helpful. In a study reported in the August 1995 issue of *Sleep*, such devices help about 60 percent of people who have obstructive sleep apnea.

➤ *Try a "snore alarm."* At least one company (Sharper Image) sells a wrist-watch that monitors snoring and wakes you up with a silent alarm consisting of powerful vibrations that begin as soon as you start to snore.

No matter what, it's important that you don't give up when it comes to finding a solution to your snoring problem. If you consistently snore and suffer signs of sleep deprivation, get yourself to a doctor for an evaluation. If you're diagnosed with sleep apnea, persevere until you find a treatment that works for you. Not only will your bed partner thank you for giving him or her the chance for consistent good sleep, but you'll be helping to significantly improve your general health as well as your daytime alertness levels.

We hope these suggestions help you—and your partner—get a better night's sleep. In the next chapter, we discuss another set of sleep disorders—including sleep walking and talking, teeth grinding, and two related syndromes called Restless Leg Movement Disorder and Periodic Leg Movement Disorder—that also disrupt sleep.

The Least You Need to Know

➤ Snoring and sleep apnea are the most common—and most undertreated—sleep problems in the United States today.

➤ Obstructive Sleep Apnea is a very common but very serious medical condition that requires medical treatment.

➤ Help for snorers and their partners does exist!

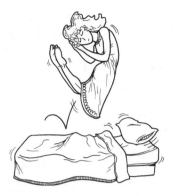

Chapter 15

When You Can't Sleep Still

In This Chapter

➤ Restless Leg Syndrome and Periodic Limb Movement Disorder

➤ The sleep "paranormals": night terrors, sleepwalking, sleeptalking, and REM behavior disorder

➤ Ways to enjoy quiet, still nights of sleep

A swift kick to the calf, the sound of grinding teeth, the thought that a child might wander out of bed into a dangerous situation—these and other nighttime events disturb the sleep of millions of people throughout the world. If you or someone in your household experiences such events, you're far from alone.

In Chapter 1, we described the common characteristics of sleep, and two of them concerned posture: When you sleep you're usually lying down and, except for occasionally changing your sleep position, you're usually lying *still*.

In the group of sleep disorders we discuss in this chapter, however, the people affected aren't able to sleep in stillness. Instead, they experience one of a number of disruptive sleep behaviors usually just as disturbing to bed partners and other household members as it is to themselves. Finding a way to alleviate or eliminate these behaviors becomes an important goal for everyone involved.

Shake, Rattle, and Roll

Two separate conditions, Restless Leg Syndrome and Periodic Limb Movement Disorder, involve convulsive movements that disturb sleep. They represent two distinct disorders, however, each with a different set of symptoms and solutions.

As its name suggests, Restless Leg Syndrome (RLS) affects primarily the legs, although it can involve the arms as well. Practically everyone with the disorder describes the symptoms in slightly different way, but it boils down to a "creepy-crawly," almost painful feeling in their legs that usually occurs when they're sitting or lying still. For some, RLS is very painful, but the pain is not like the kind that comes with a leg cramp or like the feeling of numbness that comes from a lack of oxygen supply to the leg. It most often involves a tingling or uncomfortable feeling in the calves that you can temporarily relieve by stretching or moving your legs.

Although RLS occurs while you're awake, it can also affect the quantity and quality of your sleep. The constant need to stretch or move the legs to shake free of the discomfort often prevents you from falling or staying asleep. As a result, you may become sleep deprived and suffer excess daytime sleepiness. RLS may further interfere with your lifestyle because you may not be able to sit still for any length of time, cutting short the time you can comfortably travel or participate in other activities (such as attending a play or movie) that require sitting still.

Treatment for Restless Leg Syndrome consists of both home remedies and, in more severe and stubborn cases, drug therapy. Many sufferers find that taking a hot bath, massaging the affected leg, or applying a heating pad or ice pack to the leg helps alleviate the symptoms. Taking aspirin or other pain relievers and avoiding caffeine also may help, as can getting regular exercise. Since anemia and iron defficiency are causes of RLS, taking supplemental iron pills can help.

When such home remedies fail and sleep is regularly disrupted, a doctor may prescribe a benzodiazapine (an anti-anxiety medication) or a drug commonly used to treat Parkinson's disease (L-dopa or bromocriptine, for example).

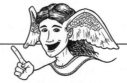

Morpheus Says

You know that feeling you get when you're startled out of sleep, as if you've just fallen off a curb? Or have you felt your leg or arm jerk quickly, just once, for no apparent reason while you're trying to fall asleep? These symptoms are called hypnic jerks, and they represent a totally harmless body reflex that wakes you as you fall asleep. Hypnic jerks involve the temporary disruption in the part of the nervous system that controls your sense of balance and are unrelated to RLS or other sleep disorders.

Periodic Limb Movement Disorder (PLMD), on the other hand, is involuntary and occurs most often when a person is fully asleep. The affected person is usually not aware of the movements.

These movements occur at regular intervals, usually every 30 seconds. They consist of a rhythmic extension of the big toe, together with an upward bending of the ankle, knee, or hip, each twitch lasting for 1 to 3 seconds. The movements are usually not continuous throughout the night, but instead cluster in the first half of the night during NREM sleep.

Doctors diagnose PLMD when the leg movements occur five or more times during each hour of sleep. The movements themselves appear to do no damage, and some good sleepers don't suffer from sleep deprivation or other problems because of them. However, if the twitches are strong, or if they occur in a light sleeper, they can actually wake them up. Needless to say, a main symptom of PLMD may be excess daytime sleepiness for both those who suffer from the disorder and for their bed partners.

Unless PLMD is severe enough to disrupt your, or your partner's, sleep on a regular basis, no treatment is recommended. In some cases, doctors will prescribe the same medications used for treating Restless Leg Syndrome. Unfortunately, no home remedies have been found to alleviate the problem.

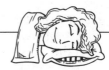

Sleep on it

If your bed partner suffers from RLS or PLMD—or any parasomnia for that matter—you may want to sleep alone in another bed until the problem is alleviated. Otherwise, your sleep is likely to be disturbed as much or even more than that of your partner.

The Sleep "Paranormal"

Parasomnias are a group of conditions or behaviors that occur during, or are exacerbated by, sleep. The most common type of parasomnias are called "disorders of arousal," and include sleepwalking, sleeptalking, night terrors, and REM behavior disorder.

Experts believe the various types of arousal disorders are related and share some characteristics, including the following:

➤ Arousal usually occurs during slow-wave (Stages 3 and 4) sleep.

➤ Body movement usually takes place.

➤ Mental confusion and disorientation are present.

➤ Difficulty achieving full wakefulness occurs, along with an impaired response to external stimuli.

➤ There is difficulty recalling the episode.

These arousals generally occur when a person is in a mixed state of sleep and wakefulness, usually coming out of the deepest stages of non-dreaming sleep. Parasomnias are very common in young children, and often pass with normal development. They may persist, however, or arise for the first time later in life. Such disorders tend to run in families. Let's take a look at the different types and see what we know about why and how they occur, and what you can do to resolve them.

Night Terrors

Night terrors (also called "sleep terrors") are the most extreme and dramatic form of arousal disorders. A night terror episode usually begins with a bloodcurdling scream or shout. Individuals experiencing night terrors have been known to bolt out of bed, run out of the house, even do harm to themselves or others. Their pupils are dilated, they're sweating profusely, their heart rates are elevated, and they're generally terrified. Unlike nightmares, however, night terrors occur without dream recall—those who experience them have no idea what frightens them so terribly. Sometimes the sleeper wakes without any memory at all of having been frightened or of screaming. Needless to say, night terrors are most disturbing for both those who experience them and for their bed partners and housemates.

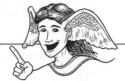

Morpheus Says

In most cases of arousal disorders in children, there's no need to worry or even to consult a doctor. However, contact your doctor if your child experiences disturbed sleep that causes:

➤ Potentially dangerous behavior that is violent or may result in injury

➤ Extreme disturbance to other household members

➤ Excessive sleepiness during the day

No one knows what causes night terrors, although a disruption in the nervous system appears to be involved. As is true for other parasomnias, night terrors are fairly common in children, especially those between the ages of 5 and 7. Kids tend to outgrow the problem naturally, without treatment. Only about 1 percent of adults develop this disorder. In susceptible people, stress, sleep deprivation, or even just sleeping in a strange bed can trigger an episode of night terror. Medication, regular exercise, and adequate sleep are the most common treatments for night terrors in adults.

Walking After Midnight

Although most common in children between the ages of 6 and 12, sleepwalking can also plague adults. In fact, according to the American Medical Association, some four million Americans have sought help for sleepwalking, also known as *somnambulism*. Sleepwalking usually takes place in the first third of the night and most often involves simple walking or other repetitive movement. Remarkably, a sleepwalker is often able to safely negotiate around objects and furniture.

Usually, the episodes last only a few minutes before the individual returns to normal sleep. It is usually best not to try to wake a sleepwalker; instead, simply help them back to bed and let them wake up on their own. Nightmares, bedwetting, and night terrors can also occur in those who sleepwalk, especially children. Interestingly enough, an EEG of a person sleepwalking shows a mixture of sleep and wake activity—in other words, a sleepwalker truly is half asleep and half awake.

Fever, sleep deprivation, or emotional upset can trigger sleepwalking. If you or your partner sleepwalks, it's important for you to seek medical advice. No one knows exactly what causes sleepwalking, but extreme stress, worry, and—rarely—a brain disorder like epilepsy may cause the disturbance. In some cases, medication like Valium, Tofranil, and even some stimulants have helped to alleviate sleepwalking.

Night Owl Wisdom

Somnabulism, or sleepwalking, is a parasomnia that involves walking about and performing other actions in a semiautomatic way during sleep without later memory of having done so.

Wake Up!

Although it's unlikely that you'll do anything to hurt yourself or others while sleepwalking, you could fall down a flight of stairs or walk outside into traffic. To avoid such danger, sleep on the first floor, keep all doors locked, and hide the keys to the car!

Acting Out Your Dreams

As you may remember from Chapter 3, your muscles become virtually paralyzed when you enter REM sleep—the stage of sleep in which you dream. This is a good thing, for otherwise we'd all be acting out our dreams in the middle of the night, without being conscious of our behavior.

Unfortunately, for some people, that's exactly what happens. For reasons as yet poorly understood, people who suffer from *REM behavior disorder* (RBD)—mostly older males— truly act out their dreams. In one case, reported by Dr. James Maas in his book *Power Sleep* (Villard, 1998), a British man shot his new bride to death while he dreamt of being pursued by gangsters. According the *Encyclopedia of Sleep and Dreaming*, people with RBD do not act out "normal" dreams, but instead carry out distinctly abnormal and often violent dreams. Interestingly enough, they are rarely the aggressor in these dreams, but instead are acting out their efforts to protect themselves or their loved ones from an attacker.

Indeed, RBD is a serious medical problem that can result in injury and death if left untreated. Over 75 percent of RBD patients have sustained repeated injuries such as bruises, lacerations requiring stitches, and fractures. Their bed partners are almost equally at risk; one woman, for instance, sustained three broken ribs from a single punch delivered by her sleeping husband.

No one knows what causes REM behavior disorder, but it appears that the muscles never receive the "paralysis" message from the cluster of cells in the brain stem responsible for this function. Doctors treat REM behavior disorder with medications such as clonazepam (Klonopin), a tranquilizer that is part of the class of drugs known as benzodiazepines.

Night Owl Wisdom

REM behavior disorder (RBD) is a parasomnia in which you act out part of a dream. Thought to be due to a malfunction in the brain stem cells that normally inhibit all muscle tone in REM sleep, this disorder can result in bizarre and disruptive behavior.

Grind Those Teeth

No one who has ever heard it will ever forget the sound made by teeth as they grind together, the raw edge of it, the spine-tingling, nerve-shattering rasp of it. An estimated one in 20 adults and three in 20 children unconsciously grind their teeth, disturbing those around them and putting themselves at risk for serious dental trouble.

The grinding of teeth during sleep, called *bruxism*, is a very common occurrence and usually isn't associated with any significant medical or psychological problems. However, severe bruxism may be associated with sleep disruption and sleep deprivation. In addition, nocturnal grinding can exert thousands of pounds of pressure per square inch on teeth surfaces. It not only can damage the teeth, but also the bone, the gums, and the jaw joint.

Night Owl Wisdom

Bruxism is a habit that involves grinding one's teeth, particularly during sleep.

Until recently, doctors attributed bruxism to the release of tension from emotional stress. However, many dental authorities today believe that the cause is related to an unconscious effort to correct irregularities of the chewing surfaces of the teeth. Dentists term such irregularities malocclusions. Simply put, people who grind their teeth may be doing so in order to find a comfortable place to fit the upper and lower teeth together.

If you or someone you love has this nightly grind problem, your first stop should be your dentist's office. The dentist may recommend using a plastic device (mouth guard); although a mouth guard does not reduce the amount of grinding, it can be quite helpful in preventing damage to the teeth. It also mutes the grinding sound that could be disturbing your or your partner's sleep.

Solutions for a Better Tomorrow

In almost all cases of sleep disorders and parasomnias, the better you sleep, and the less sleep deprived you are, the less likely you'll be to suffer their symptoms. That means you should review all of the chapters in Part 2 for hints on improving your sleep hygiene. That means examining your dietary habits, reducing caffeine intake, staying away from too much alcohol before bedtime, exercising regularly, finding ways to reduce and relieve stress, and creating a sleep-friendly environment in your bedroom.

In this chapter, we discussed one general category of sleep disorders involving inappropriate behavior and movement. Next, we examine what happens when your sleep comes at the wrong time and, in some cases, in the wrong place.

The Least You Need to Know

➤ Restless Leg Syndrome and Periodic Limb Movement Disorder are common and treatable conditions.

➤ While sleepwalking and sleeptalking are often harmless, night terrors and REM behavior disorders may be more dangerous. However, all will benefit from a medical evaluation if sleep deprivation develops.

➤ Practicing good sleep hygiene will lessen the symptoms of all sleep disorders.

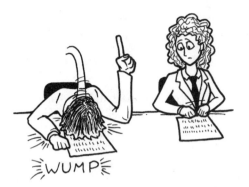

Chapter 16

The Wrong Place, the Wrong Time

> ### In This Chapter
>
> ➤ The signs and symptoms of narcolepsy
>
> ➤ Understanding circadian rhythms disorders
>
> ➤ Sleep well—at the right time and place

Nothing feels better than slipping into bed at the end of a long day, descending into sleep, then waking up hours later ready to meet the new day. Sleep is a good thing.

But try telling that to those people—and there are millions of them—who, for one reason or another, take their sleep at the wrong time, whose "hardwiring" has somehow gone haywire. In this chapter, we discuss two separate types of problems related to the timing of sleep: First, we'll explore a disorder in which a person experiences such severe daytime sleepiness that he or she falls asleep suddenly at any time of the day. Then, we'll show you the world of the "circadian-disturbed"—those people whose body clocks are set so far off the "average" that it significantly interferes with their ability to function day-to-day.

If you suffer from any of these conditions, or know someone who does, read on for information and advice.

What Is Narcolepsy?

No doubt there have been days when you've felt so tired that it feels like you could fall asleep standing up—everybody has felt like this at some point or another. However, in some cases, such a condition is chronic and debilitating. Called *narcolepsy*, this condition affects approximately one in 1,000 people in the United States, just about the same number affected by multiple sclerosis or Parkinson's disease. According to the National Sleep Foundation, about 250,000 Americans suffer from narcolepsy.

Defining Narcolepsy

The word *narcolepsy* comes from the Greek *narke*, for "numbness," and *lambanein*, which means "to seize." Narcolepsy is a neurological sleep disorder that essentially involves an attack of REM sleep—the dreaming portion of sleep—during the day. It is characterized by excessive daytime sleepiness, cataplexy, sleep paralysis, and hypnagogic hallucinations—terms we explain in more detail later in this chapter.

Night Owl Wisdom

Narcolepsy is a neurological sleep disorder that causes irresistible sleepiness during the day.

Narcolepsy can begin at any age and often continues throughout life. It often becomes noticeable during the teens or early twenties, but can also first appear later in life. There seems to be genetic connection: Close relatives of people with narcolepsy are 60 times more likely to suffer from the disorder than are members of the general population.

A person with narcolepsy has recurring episodes of lapses into sleep. These lapses can last anywhere from several seconds to 10 to 20 minutes. You wake up from this "nap" feeling refreshed for an hour or two until drowsiness returns. Called "sleep attacks," these sudden sleep episodes can occur in awkward and even dangerous situations, and often without warning.

Night Owl Wisdom

HLA-DR2 is a part of a class of gene products expressed on cell surfaces, including leukocytes (white blood cells). HLA stands for human leukocyte antigen.

As you may remember from Chapter 3, REM sleep begins after you've passed through the first four stages of sleep. With narcolepsy, REM sleep starts almost immediately. Since the brain may not be totally asleep when dreaming begins, the dream is sometimes experienced more vividly and is thought of as an hallucination. These REM periods, or fragments of them, occur inappropriately during the day.

The exact cause of narcolepsy is not clearly understood. It appears to be a biological problem, possibly involving abnormalities of brain chemistry. It often runs in families; geneticists have found a remarkable association between narcolepsy and the presence of a specific group of genes called *HLA-DR2*.

The Symptoms

The symptoms of narcolepsy are usually first noticed during teenage or young adult years, although it can strike at any age. Different individuals experience wide variations in both the development, the number, and the severity of their symptoms. The primary symptoms of narcolepsy include:

➤ *Excessive daytime sleepiness, often so severe that the sufferer falls asleep unexpectedly many times a day.* Persistent drowsiness that may continue for prolonged periods of time and microsleeps—fleeting moments of sleep intruding into the waking state—may also occur. Not only is this condition embarrassing, it can also be very dangerous.

➤ *Muscle weakness when emotions are strong.* Called *cataplexy*, this symptom involves sudden loss of muscle function ranging from slight weakness (such as limpness of the neck or knees, sagging facial muscles, or an inability to speak clearly) to complete body collapse. The person remains conscious throughout the episode, which may last from a few seconds to several minutes. One of the most striking features of cataplexy is its association with specific situations or emotions. The most common triggers are laughter, anger, surprise, and excitement.

➤ *Inability to move for several minutes after waking up.* Called sleep paralysis (we first described this in Chapter 2), this problem is related to the disruption of REM sleep.

➤ *Vivid, realistic, often frightening dreams.* Also called hypnagogic hallucinations, these intense experiences occur at the beginning or end of the sleep period. Often the person has the sensation of being paralyzed and then perceives some threatening figure or event nearby.

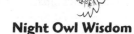

Night Owl Wisdom

A symptom of narcolepsy, **cataplexy** is the sudden attack of complete or partial muscular paralysis, often precipitated by a strong emotion.

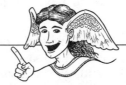

Morpheus Says

Hypnagogic hallucinations may also involve auditory signs consisting of simple repetitive sounds or involving complex musical themes. In one study of narcolepsy, a patient reported hearing a scratched record playing the same sentence over and over again during his hypnagogic episodes. The hallucinations themselves usually consist of a meaningful and dramatic visual sequence that forms a story or part of a story.

The Diagnosis

If your doctor suspects narcolepsy based on a description of your symptoms, he or she will probably suggest that you visit a sleep laboratory for an evaluation. There, you'll be hooked up to a polysomnograph to measure your sleep patterns during the day and during the night. A diagnosis of narcolepsy is made if the polysomnograph shows one or both of the following:

➤ Falling asleep in under 10 minutes during the day.

➤ REM sleep occurring in less than 20 minutes.

Wake Up!

If you've experienced a recent dramatic change in your sleep/wake patterns or a major life stressor (the death of a relative, a divorce, a big move) and suddenly feel overwhelmed by sleep during the day, ask your doctor about narcolepsy—especially if you don't think you're having trouble sleeping at night. Some research suggests that the initial symptoms of narcolepsy may follow abrupt changes of the sleep/wake schedule or an emotional trauma.

Living with Narcolepsy

People living with narcolepsy often develop psychological problems due to the difficulty they have both with coping with the symptoms and coping with other people's reaction to the disorder. It's often very hard for someone with narcolepsy—and the people around him or her—to accept the fact that sleepiness and sleep attacks are uncontrollable and that the person isn't lazy or irresponsible. Failure to accept this fact may negatively influence self-esteem and personal relationships.

Although narcolepsy does not directly affect intelligence, it may disrupt an affected person's education. Concentration, memory, and attention may be periodically impaired by drowsiness and sleep. Children with narcolepsy should be identified at the earliest possible age to avoid developing a pattern of failure and feelings of low self-esteem.

People with narcolepsy can and do lead productive lives—indeed, people with narcolepsy work in every kind of job and career imaginable—as long as they receive proper medical care. Parents, teachers, spouses, and employers must be made aware of the symptoms of narcolepsy so that they won't make the mistake of confusing such behavior with laziness, hostility, rejection, or lack of interest and motivation. Once an employer understands, he or she may be able to help by providing the time and space someone with narcolepsy needs to take scheduled naps and work breaks. In fact, under the Americans with Disabilities Act (ADA), an employer is required by law to make reasonable accommodations for those with narcolepsy in the workplace.

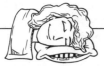

Sleep on it

Narcoleptic symptoms may appear as early as age 10, which means school problems may result. Schools *must* provide extra help for your child under the Individuals with Disabilities Education Act (IDEA). Talk to the principal, guidance counselor, or school administrator if you have any questions.

Stay-Awake Solutions

The goal of treatment for narcolepsy is to keep you as alert as possible during the day and to minimize any recurring episodes of cataplexy. Your doctor will probably recommend one or more of the following treatments:

➤ *Medication.* The main treatment of excessive daytime sleepiness in narcolepsy is with a group of drugs called central nervous system stimulants. They include dextroamphetamine sulfate (Dexedrine), methylphenidate hydrocholoride (Ritalin), and pemoline (Cylert). For cataplexy and other REM-sleep symptoms, antidepressant medication and other drugs that suppress REM sleep are pre-scribed. One category includes imipramine (Tofranil), desimipramine (Norpramin), and clomipramine (Anafranil). Selective serotonin re-uptake inhibi-tors (SSRIs) such as fluoxetine (Prozac) and paroxetine (Paxil) may also be helpful. A new wake-promoting drug called modafinil (Provigil) is currently under review by the Food and Drug Administration for use in the United States.

➤ *Scheduled naps.* An important part of treat-ment is scheduled short naps of about 10 to 15 minutes each, two to three times a day. Such naps help to control daytime sleepiness and keep you as alert as possible.

➤ *Avoidance of alcohol.* As you know from past chapters, drinking alcohol can disrupt your sleep—and that's just as true for those who suffer from narcolepsy.

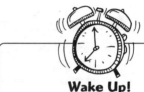

Wake Up!

If you're pregnant or thinking about becoming pregnant and take medication to treat your narcolepsy, talk to your doctor about the possible effects of the medication on the fetus.

Narcolepsy is one kind of sleep disorder that has you sleeping when you'd rather be awake. Those who suffer from circadian rhythm disorders find themselves in the same situation, though these conditions have very different symptoms, causes, and treatments.

Lark Songs and Owl Hoots

As we've already discussed at length, some people are Larks, which means that they just naturally prefer to get up early in the morning and retire early in the evening. Others we call Owls, because they just naturally like going to bed late at night and sleeping later into the morning.

In most cases, these simple preferences are easy to manage. Although it may be slightly more difficult for a Lark to stay up past midnight, and an Owl may struggle with having to attend an early morning meeting, both types usually can adapt fairly easily, especially if they practice good sleep hygiene and make other accommodations to their daily schedules.

For a small percentage of the population, however, there is a misalignment between their internal clocks and the "normal" sleep/wake pattern followed by most of society. In other words, they have biological clocks that keep them awake and put them to sleep at times that are extremely disruptive to their lives. In some cases, they fall asleep and get up way too early; in others, they go to bed and get up way too late.

It's important to note that these disorders, which we describe in the following sections, do not interfere with the ability to sleep or the quality of sleep. If real life didn't intrude, these people would be perfectly happy and well, waking and sleeping according to their own patterns. But the world—of school, work, family, life—*does* intrude, and they're left trying to deny their own rhythms for the sake of living in step with the rest of us. Fortunately, there are ways for them to reset the clock, at least enough to make ordinary daily living possible.

DSPS: The Late Show

Although many of us in this chronically sleep deprived society love to stay up late and "sleep in" as much as our lives allow, some among us suffer from a distinct sleep disorder that makes it almost impossible to go to bed and get up during "regular" hours.

Delayed Sleep Phase Syndrome (DSPS), for instance, is a fairly common disorder of sleep timing. People with DSPS tend to fall asleep at very late times, and also have difficulty waking up in time for normal work, school, or social needs. Typically, the affected person is unable to fall asleep until 3 or 4 a.m. or later and finds it difficult or impossible to sustain alertness during the day if they have to wake before 10 or 11 a.m. If they are forced to rise at 7 a.m. or so to go to a 9-to-5 job or to school, they become seriously sleep deprived—but even then cannot fall asleep until 3 or 4 a.m.

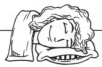

Sleep on it

It is very important to determine if your teenager's inability to get up in the morning and stay awake and alert at school results from normal changes in sleep patterns, a clinical sleep disorder like DSPS, or is related to depression or another problem, such as a learning disability. Talk to your doctor if you have concerns.

Because body temperature and other circadian rhythms also tend to "run late" in people with DSPS, it is likely that the disorder results from an abnormality in the timing mechanism that governs sleep and wakefulness. In some cases, it could be that these people are not as sensitive to light cues as others, and therefore cannot depend on the prime Zeitgeber of sunlight to maintain their internal clock. In others, their natural body clock may run with a cycle of longer than 25 hours, causing a delay in the onset of normal sleep periods.

The disorder often first appears in late childhood and adolescence. In fact, some studies indicate that as many as 15 to 20 percent of university students may be affected, though their symptoms tend to be discounted as simply a side-effect of puberty. Once established, the condition often persists for many years and may be more severe in the autumn and winter months.

As we discuss in Chapter 20, many teenagers naturally tend to want to sleep late in the morning and go to bed late at night. Most will grow out of this tendency as they enter their 20s. However, there are some who suffer from DSPS, but never receive a proper diagnosis. These people usually blame themselves—or their families blame them—thinking that they're simply lazy and unmotivated. To counter this assumption, those with DSPS often force themselves to get up on time, by the use of multiple alarm clocks if necessary, and then struggle through the day on only two or three hours of sleep. Despite their exhaustion, however, they are often unable to fall asleep before the wee hours of the morning.

Needless to say, those with DSPS are likely to gravitate toward the night shift and/or to occupations with late working hours (the restaurant and entertainment industries, for instance) or flexible ones (self-employed writers, free-lance computer programmers, etc.). They are the direct opposites of their extreme Lark counterparts who suffer from a disorder called Advanced Sleep Phase Syndrome (ASPS).

ASPS: The Way-Too Early Bird

Far less common than DSPS, ASPS is a disorder in which the major sleep episode is advanced in relation to the desired clock time. This mistiming results in symptoms of compelling evening sleepiness, an early sleep onset, and an awakening that is earlier than desired, often before dawn. Typically, sleep onset occurs between 6 p.m. and 9 p.m. and wake-up before 5 a.m., sometimes as early as 1 a.m.—making those with ASPS the worst dinner dates imaginable!

In contrast to DSPS, in which teenagers and young adults are most affected, ASPS most frequently affects middle-aged and older people. In fact, as we'll discuss further in Chapter 22, early awakening is a normal part of the aging process and ASPS may represent an excessive expression of this tendency. Like their counterparts, those with ASPS get a normal quantity and quality of sleep—when they're able to set their own schedules. Otherwise, they often become sleep deprived as they go without sleep in order to live in the "real" world.

Resetting Your Clock

Both DSPS and ASPS respond well to two often related treatments. The first is chronotherapy, in which—with help from experts at a sleep lab or on their own with guidance—the patients force themselves to go to bed a few hours later (in the case of DSPS) or earlier (in the case of ASPS) every day until they achieve their desired bedtime by progressively moving sleep time around the clock. This process can take up to two weeks, but is often successful. The trick, however, is that once they achieve this new, acceptable bedtime, they must NEVER deviate from it, or they'll have to start the resetting process all over again. Remember, DSPS and ASPS are disorders of the internal clock, a clock that clearly runs on its own time.

One particularly helpful adjunct to chronotherapy is bright light therapy, which we discussed in some depth in Chapter 11. Those with DSPS can move their biological clocks forward eastward by exposing themselves to daylight first thing in the morning and avoiding bright light in the evening. People with ASPS reset their internal clocks by exposing themselves to bright light during the late evening hours, and making sure to keep their bedrooms pitch black during the early morning hours. Adding a dose of melatonin, a hormone that helps set the stage for sleep, an hour or two before the appropriate bedtime can also help both types of sleep-disordered people reset their body clocks and get a good night's sleep.

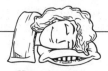

Sleep on it

If you suffer from DSPS, you may want to talk to your doctor about taking extra doses of vitamin B12. Some studies show that this vitamin helps increase your sensitivity to bright light, thereby helping to reset your clock for earlier sleep and wake-up times.

The problem of sleeping at the wrong time and the wrong place is not limited to those with sleep disorders. People who work the night shift, for instance, also have to sleep when their bodies tell them to be awake and must stay alert and active when they'd rather go to sleep. This is the subject we take up in the next chapter. Another group of people whose rhythms become disrupted are those who travel across time zones. You'll learn about that challenge in Chapter 18.

The Least You Need to Know

➤ Falling asleep during the day may be a sign not of sleep deprivation but of narcolepsy, a serious sleep disorder.

➤ Treatment, including medication and scheduled napping, can help those with narcolepsy enjoy safe and productive lives.

➤ Disorders of the circadian clock disturb the lives of millions of people, but careful treatment can help them reset their internal clocks to "normal" time.

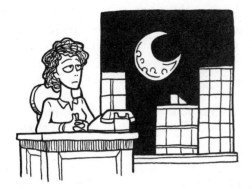

Chapter 17

The Night Shift

In This Chapter

➤ The world of night work

➤ Understanding the effects of working nights

➤ Learning to make the best of a tough work schedule

A 24-hour society…that's pretty much the state of the world as we speed headlong into the 21st century. There are fast becoming very few limits to the activities we can perform at any hour of the day almost anywhere in the world.

For millions of years, however, our ancestors have awakened with the sun and slept after dark, and because of our intrinsic, biological need for sleep at night, most of us still go to bed around 11 p.m. and get up by 7 a.m. (give or take an hour or two at each end). We prefer to sleep at this time because our bodies are primed to do so by the internal timekeeper known as the biological clock.

But things are different for the 20 million Americans who work the night shift and the millions of caregivers of loved ones who need attention around the clock. These people must resist their natural instincts and stay up when they should be asleep. And not only must they simply remain awake, but they also have to function at high levels, performing sensitive tasks that require coordination and thought. Although an occasional night of sleeplessness may cause some temporary discomfort, working the night shift over the long haul may disrupt a wide range of biological rhythms, which can lead to a variety of potentially serious psychological and physical symptoms.

In this chapter, we discuss the world of night work and the physical problems it can cause. We also offer you some tips on how to better deal with the stress that night work puts on your body and soul. We do so from two angles. First, we'll help you get through the night when you're feeling sleep-deprived, then we'll show you how to manage over the long haul with tips on how to improve your general health habits and get as much sleep as possible on a regular basis.

Working Yourself to Death

It's important to know right from the start that unless you're one of the lucky few extreme Owls who naturally thrive at night or you learn to reset your biological clock by judicious use of light and other methods, your body simply won't "get used" to working when it otherwise would be sleeping.

At the very least, the side effects of working at night are uncomfortable. They not only can have a negative impact on your general health, they can also disrupt your family and social life. The level of disruption night work causes depends both on how flexible your body is to changes in schedule and the type of shift you work. In fact, there are several types of shift work schedules—rotating shifts; fixed 8,10, and 12-hour shifts; evening shifts; night shifts; and thousands of variations of these shifts—each with its own set of advantages, disadvantages, and side effects. Because it goes far beyond the scope of this book to discuss specifics of each shift work type, we'll focus on some of the most common and more general problems caused by working at night on a regular basis.

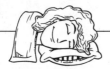

Sleep on it

To find out how well you'd adapt to shift work, ask yourself how long you can sleep during the day after an "all-nighter." If you can sleep for seven or eight hours, you may do well. Then ask yourself how well you handle jet lag. The ability to bounce back from a six-hour time change within a day or two indicates that you may be a good candidate for shift work.

Before we get started, we do want to reiterate that some people actually thrive on the night shift. Natural Owls, for instance, find themselves attracted to this lifestyle because it suits their innate tendency to function best at night. Some Regular Robins can adapt easily and well to working at night, and also enjoy the freedom of having the afternoons off that such a schedule permits.

Nevertheless, many night workers find themselves plagued with symptoms and side effects—medical and social—resulting from the disruption of circadian rhythms.

The Medical Downside

As you know by now, your body has its own internal schedule, one that keeps you alert and awake during the day and asleep at night. Whenever you disrupt this rhythm—due to jet lag, night work, or a sleep disorder—you risk developing some related medical problems, some minor, others more serious. Here are some of the most common:

➤ *Mood and memory problems.* Just one night of missed sleep can make you cranky and forgetful, so you can imagine what running at a near-constant sleep debt does to your psychological stability! A few studies suggest that shift work may be linked to depression. A study of Italian textile workers, for instance, found that night workers reported a far higher incidence of anxiety or depression requiring treatment than day workers.

➤ *Sleep deprivation.* Over time, the average night worker obtains about two hours less sleep a day than the average nine-to-fiver. One study reported that between one- and two-thirds of night workers report that they fall asleep at least once a week on the job. In addition, according to the American Sleep Disorders Association, five million people suffer from sleep deprivation as a result of shift work.

➤ *Possible increased risk of infection.* A 1996 study in the *Journal of Experimental Biology* found that people forced to stay up later than usual showed a decrease in the activity of *natural killer cells*, immune system blood cells that fight disease.

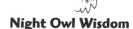

Night Owl Wisdom

Natural killer cells, often abbreviated NK, are immune system cells that form a line of defense against infection. When you lose sleep, your body fails to produce its usual supply of these cells, which could leave you more vulnerable to infection.

➤ *Gastrointestinal disorders.* Numerous studies show that working nights raises an employee's risk of developing a variety of gastrointestinal problems, including ulcers, bowel irregularities (constipation or diarrhea), excessive gas, abdominal pain, and heartburn. Shift work is hard on the stomach for a number of reasons that include lack of sleep, disruption of circadian rhythms, poor eating habits, excess coffee and alcohol consumption, smoking, and stress.

➤ *Cardiovascular disease.* The general consensus is that shift work raises an individual's risk of developing heart disease by 30 to 50 percent, even after accounting for lifestyle factors such as smoking and diet. That makes it less of a risk than smoking cigarettes or being obese, for instance, but still a significant problem.

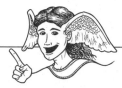

Morpheus Says

The connection between shift work and heart disease may involve several factors. The disruption to circadian rhythms may increase blood pressure and blood cholesterol levels, both of which contribute to the development of heart disease. The high stress levels experienced by shift workers also add to the risk. Studies also show that shift workers are more likely than day workers to lead sedentary lives, be overweight, and consume high-fat diets, all risk factors for heart disease.

➤ *Reproductive risks.* Some studies suggest that shift work can affect a woman's ability to get pregnant and carry a fetus to term. A European study, for instance, found that women shift workers on rotating schedules experience conception delays of more than nine months when they try to conceive. A British study found that shift work increased the risk of miscarriage by 44 percent, while a French study found that shift work increased the risk of premature births by 60 percent.

As startling as these statistics about the effect working nights has on your health are, it's important to keep them in perspective. First of all, just because there is an increased risk across the population doesn't mean that you, as an individual, will suffer such an increase. Second, shift work ranks near the bottom of the list of avoidable risk factors: Smoking, obesity, and lack of exercise are far more important in the development of heart disease, for instance, than shift work. Finally, there is still much to be learned about the effects of shift work on health, and the conclusions reached in the studies we cite here may or may not be modified as we learn more.

Equally variable are the effects of shift work on family relationships. Some families adjust quite well, especially if they structure their time wisely and plan family activities with care. Others have more difficulty, as you'll see in the next section.

The Social Stresses

As practically any American adult can tell you today, balancing work and family life is a demanding responsibility even in the easiest of circumstances. Add to it the challenges posed by shift work, and you may have a recipe for familial discord and miscommunication. In fact, studies show that the divorce rate in shift-working families is 60 percent higher than for day workers. Indeed, the stresses on family life when one or both parents work around the clock or have irregular schedules are great:

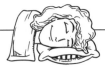

Sleep on it

Take advantage of on-site, 24-hour child care. Some companies now offer round-the-clock day care for children of employees who work the night shift. Taking advantage of such a benefit can help reduce the stress surrounding your child-care issues.

➤ *The absent parent.* Needless to say, shift work makes it more difficult than ever to spend time with your children. The evening shift (usually 4 p.m. to midnight) may be the toughest, since you leave for work before your children return from school and get home after they're in bed. And if you and your spouse both work shifts, the chances that your children will get all the attention they need from you are even more remote.

➤ *Family stress.* You're tired and cranky when you get home from a 12-hour shift, but your spouse and children crave your attention. Instead of giving it to them, you crawl into bed and throw the covers over your head for hours. When you wake up, the last thing you want to do is fix a family meal or repair the broken lawn mower (which you promised to do a week ago). Resentment can build, and build quickly, among all family members.

As you can see, working nights can disrupt many aspects of your life if you're not careful. Later in the chapter, we'll offer some tips on how to make the best of your time off, including how to get the sleep you need to protect your health as much as possible.

In the meantime, let's discuss another challenge for many people who work the night shift: Making it through the long nights awake and alert when your body would much rather be asleep.

Getting Through the Night: The Short Term

With any luck, you'll be one of the few who adapt well to shift work, which means that you'll be able to get the sleep you need during the day and thus avoid becoming sleep deprived. Even so, you may have trouble making it through the entire night without experiencing a dip in energy and concentration at some point during your shift, particularly in the early morning hours.

In Chapter 13, we outlined some of the ways you can help your body feel more alert and focused, suggestions that certainly bear repeating here, along with a few others more specifically targeted to the shift worker, including:

➤ *Come to work rested.* We know that's easier said than done, which is why we give you some tips on how to sleep during the day later in the chapter. But simply put, the more sleep you get, the better you'll be able to accommodate the demands on your body and mind made during the nights you must stay awake. Getting an uninterrupted night's sleep or learning to nap efficiently can help you maintain a proper sleep balance.

➤ *Vary your tasks.* If possible, take a break from the more repetitive tasks involved in your job and turn to ones that require either more intellectual creativity or more physical energy. The change in pace, along with the new demand on your attention, will help to wake you up.

➤ *Take an exercise break.* Even a short burst of exercise can help stimulate blood flow to the brain and your extremities, helping you feel more alert and refreshed. Longer bouts of exercise at night can also help you shift your circadian rhythms.

➤ *Perk up.* And yes, we mean with caffeine, judiciously ingested. By timing your use of

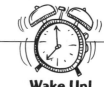

Wake Up!

Eating a large meal during your break will only make you feel sleepier. Try a bout of moderate exercise instead. Indeed, exercising late at night can help you adjust your circadian rhythms, theoretically making it easier to sleep in the daytime and stay awake at night.

caffeine, you can make it through the most difficult hours of the night without jeopardizing your sleep during the day. Although you should avoid drinking cup after cup of coffee, tea, or cola on the night shift, one or two well-timed cups will boost your alertness through the most difficult hours. Keep in mind, however, that sensitivity to caffeine varies considerably from one individual to another. Depending on your physiology, a cup of coffee early in your shift may or may not interfere with sleep when you get home. If you find it does, try substituting an ice-cold glass of water or fruit juice for coffee.

➤ *Avoid the pharmaceutical approach.* Avoid taking pharmaceutical "uppers" or sleeping pills. Their effects on your body can be dramatic and long-lasting. They can also become addictive.

➤ *Lighten up.* In Chapter 11, we discussed the profound effects of bright light on your circadian rhythms. In addition to using light to shift your clocks forward (or back, as the case may be), simply raising light levels in the work place can help you stay alert and suppress sleepiness.

➤ *Take a breath—of cool air.* Cool dry air, especially if it blows on your face, can help keep you awake and alert. Keep the room temperature cool as well, wearing a sweater if necessary for comfort.

Adapting to Night Work: The Long Haul

Although most people seem to accept the fact that some of us need to work during important social functions, they have less sympathy when you're "only" trying to sleep.

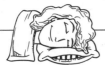

Sleep on it

Check out Circadian Technologies' Web site at www.circadian.com. This site is filled with information about circadian rhythms, sleep deprivation and its effects, and how to better cope with shiftwork physically, mentally, and socially. The site also offers a variety of pamphlets, booklets, newsletters, and other material for shiftworkers and their managers.

Indeed, it may sometimes seem as if the entire world is out to get you. Neighbors insist on mowing their lawns while you're trying to sleep. People who would never phone you at 2 a.m. (when you might just be awake!) routinely do so at 2 p.m., not understanding that they're interrupting your major sleep period.

Many studies show that those people who are most successful at shift work don't try to live in two worlds. They install answering machines, black-out curtains, and "Do Not Disturb" signs for their bedroom doors. Their friends and family know about—and respect—the importance of uninterrupted daytime sleep.

You have two basic goals here: To get enough sleep so that you stay healthy while you work shifts, and to organize your time so that your family and social life suffer as little as possible. Meeting those goals takes time and practice. We hope that some of these tips help you get started.

Optimizing Your Sleep Patterns

Finding a way to restore your body's energy and vitality when sleep comes at strange times can be a challenge. Here are a few suggestions that might help you keep your clock running in the right direction:

➤ *Split sleeping.* This is a technique that involves sleeping for several hours immediately before and several hours immediately after a night shift. Don't concern yourself with being exact about the split: The point is to get yourself two satisfying sleep periods that total the sleep you need in any 24-hour period.

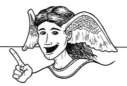

Morpheus Says

Talk about shift work: Leonardo da Vinci, a prolific and busy Renaissance man if there ever was one, spread out his sleep by taking short naps during the day. He was reputed to be active almost continuously by engaging in a 15-minute nap every four hours—giving him a total of 1.5 hours of sleep per day!

➤ *Anchor sleeping.* Anchor sleeping involves finding a time of day in which you can *always* sleep and sleeping at that time, whether you're working at night or not. Regularly taking a four-hour sleep period, say from 8 a.m. until noon, even on their days off is one way for night workers to maintain adjustment to night work. However, this approach may be difficult to pursue if you have a rotating schedule that requires you to work some mornings during this period.

➤ *Napping.* A 90-minute nap just prior to your night shift will help you remain alert and allow for better sleep when you get home. And taking a short, 15- or 20-minute nap just before you leave work will help you avoid the hazards of drowsy driving.

➤ *Understand the power of light and dark.* Remember: The sun is an important partner in your

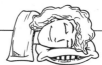

Sleep on it

If you work at night, it's especially important to take care when driving. If possible, take a short nap before you leave work to take the edge off your fatigue and sleepiness. On your way home, keep the car cool and the radio on to fight fatigue—especially if you're wearing dark sunglasses to shut out morning light in order to sleep when you get home and reset your body clock.

effort to work at night and sleep during the day. If you time your exposure to light properly, you can help shift your biological clock. Basically, if you want to stay up later at night and sleep during the morning hours, avoid light in the morning by wearing dark sunglasses on your way home, then sleeping in a dark room. Later, treat yourself to a burst of bright light in the late evening using a light visor or light box. Review Chapter 11 for more information about timing your light exposure to shift your rhythms and some of the high-tech (but afford-able) devices that can help you do so.

Making a Nest at Home

Face it: Getting the sleep you need during the day is going to be a challenge because what you really want to do is create nighttime conditions—darkness, quiet, privacy, a sense of coziness—right smack in the middle of the day. Let's see what you can do to create an environment conducive to sleep despite it all:

➤ *Stay in the dark.* Black-out curtains and blinds will help keep the daylight from streaming in your windows. Keep your door closed against ambient light from the rest of the house.

➤ *Quiet please!* Noise control is essential. Unplug the telephone in your room and place the answering machine far from where you can hear it pick up in-coming calls. Running an air conditioner can help mask noise from outside (as well as keep the air at a comfortably cool temperature, which will also help you sleep). Ask neighbors ahead of time if they could refrain from mowing their lawns or indulging in any other noisy activity during the hours you sleep.

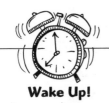

Wake Up!

Avoid turning on the television when you get home. The morning news and talk shows are far too perky and stimulating for someone who puts sleep as his or her top priority. Wait until later up to catch up on the day's events.

➤ *Aim for comfort.* Keep your bedroom at a comfort-able temperature, preferably with circulating air. Make sure your mattress and pillows support your back and head.

➤ *Establish a sleepy time routine.* Yes, it's just as important to ready your body and mind for sleep during the day as it is at night. Take a warm bath, brush your teeth, read for a little while until you feel relaxed—not exhausted, not stressed, just relaxed enough to let the pressures of your work night fade away. Then slip between the sheets and sleep.

Establishing Healthy Habits

It's more important than ever to treat your body well: You want to be as healthy as possible to endure the extra strain working at night can impose. Here are some suggestions for staying healthy:

➤ *Get regular exercise.* And the emphasis is on "regular." Being physically fit in general will help you better withstand the rigors of night work. In addition, you can use exercise like bright light exposure or anchor sleep to help you maintain or shift your body clock. Try exercising in the late afternoon, when it's still sunny out and before your next shift.

➤ *Eat well.* When you work the night shift, it may be tempting to rely on high-fat, high-sugar, quick pick-me-ups and to forget the essentials of a balanced diet. When you get home from work, it may help to eat a light meal, high in carbohydrates, such as a bowl of high-fiber cereal, which will help you sleep better. For more information about how diet affects sleep, see Chapter 7.

➤ *Take time out to relax.* It's all too easy to feel as if you have to spend every waking second doing something useful. But in order to stay healthy, you also need some downtime, when you do nothing else but relax your body and soul. Watching a videotape of last Monday night's football game is one way, practicing yoga is another. Chapter 8 provides lots of hints about reducing stress in your life.

Easing Up on Family Stress

The challenges facing a worker on the night shift go far beyond the physical: Indeed, his or her entire circle of family and friends is often affected by the demands of, and often the unpredictability of, shift work. Here are a few suggestions to help mitigate the stress:

➤ *Share schedule information.* Make sure your family members know what your work schedule is and keep them informed about any changes that occur on a daily basis. If you're facing a permanent change—from the night shift to the evening shift, for instance—you need to discuss how this change will affect the family *before* the schedule takes effect.

➤ *Keep the lines of communication open.* Keep abreast of your family's needs so that day-to-day responsibilities, such as car maintenance or child care, don't get lost in the shuffle. Even trivial matters can become major irritants if you ignore them for too long.

Sleep on it

To help you organize your time and help your family remain up-to-date about your schedule, try using Circadian Technologies' *Working Nights Family Calendar*. The calendar comes with removable color-coded stickers that help everyone, including young children, understand your schedule at a glance. You can order from our Web site at http// :www.shiftwork.com/bookstore/.

➤ *Maintain a "Family Bulletin Board."* Help everyone stay in touch by hanging up a bulletin board where you and your family can leave notes, report cards to sign, and other important messages for one another.

➤ *Plan dates for days when you're rested.* If you have trouble finding time to be alone with your partner, make a date to do something special at least once a month. When it comes to planning family outings, try to do so on days when you're likely to feel well rested, which is often not on your first day off after a week of night work. Plan carefully.

Now that you've had a chance to see how shift work can upset your biological clock—and how you can minimize its effects—it's time to examine another common activity with a similar outcome: jet lag.

The Least You Need to Know

➤ Shift work in one form or another is becoming more and more common in today's economy.

➤ Working nights can affect your health and your family life.

➤ There are techniques that can help you stay awake and alert, even when your body says it's bedtime.

➤ Making the effort to organize your time and establish healthy habits can help you stay well and optimize your chances of tolerating—and perhaps even enjoying—shift work.

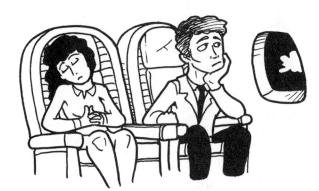

Chapter 18

Jet Lag 101

In This Chapter

➤ Exploring the world of time-zone travel

➤ Identifying the symptoms and causes of jet lag

➤ Finding solutions that work for you

What could be more exciting and stimulating to the body, mind, and spirit than hopping on a plane, flying thousands of miles through clear blue ozone, and then arriving in a completely different landscape and environment? It still seems almost magical to us naturally earthbound humans, and the pleasure and stimulation of travel would well be worth the expense and inconvenience, if only—if only!—it weren't for the jet lag, that sickly, tired, out-of-sorts feeling that overwhelms so many people as they try to adjust to a new time and place.

Fortunately, because of all that's known about the internal circadian clock, we can help you alleviate the symptoms of jet lag on your next long-distance journey, whether its for business or pleasure. Unless you're particularly hardy and a little bit lucky, you probably won't be able to eliminate jet lag entirely, but with some planning and extra care, you can make your time away from home a lot more comfortable.

The Time-Zone Rumba

It seems like a cruel trick, doesn't it? There you are, the sun shining as you munch on a croissant on the Champs Élysées in Paris or as you face potential new clients at a business meeting in Toyko—and all you can think about is getting back to bed. Maybe more sleep will stop your head from throbbing, soothe your frazzled nerves, and help you remember the name of your key contact at the meeting.

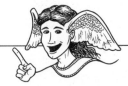

Morpheus Says

Not only can jet lag drastically reduce a tourist's simple enjoyment of a new place or the efficiency of a professional on a business trip, it can also have serious health and safety consequences. Olympic gold medalist diver Greg Louganis reported that jet lag caused the accident in which he struck his head on the 10-meter platform during a reverse dive at the 1989 Olympic trials.

And sleep would indeed help to cure your symptoms—at least in the short term. But if you were planning to spend several days or a few weeks in this new land, you'd be best served by timing your sleep very carefully right from the start. By doing so, you'd stand a better chance that—sooner rather than later—your body would catch up with the environment.

Jet Lag: Symptoms and Causes

If you've traveled across more than a few time zones, you already know the symptoms of the condition commonly known as jet lag. They include, among others:

➤ Headache

➤ Irritability

➤ Gastric discomfort

➤ Chills

➤ Difficulty with concentration

➤ Sleep problems

What you might not realize is that several different travel-related factors contribute to the development of these symptoms. Understanding each of them, and how they combine to make you feel just plain icky, may help protect you against their effects the next time you travel—and we give you tips on how to do so later in this chapter. In the meantime, it's important that you gain an understanding of just what might cause these symptoms in the first place. Among the factors influencing the development of jet lag are:

➤ *Travel fatigue.* If you've ever had to pack, get to the airport, pass through security, stand in line to check your luggage, and then wait at the stuffy gate before cramming onto a tiny, overcrowded airplane, you know just what we mean by "travel fatigue." By the time you arrive at your destination, you're more than ready for a long night's sleep in order to recover. As you'll see later, if you time it right, this state of exhaustion can actually help you in the long run.

➤ *Sleep loss.* Unless you're one of the lucky few who find it possible—even easy—to sleep on a plane, or unless your entire flight takes place during your normal daytime, you're bound to leave the plane running a sleep deficit. Again, if you're able to time your flight optimally, such a condition may work to your advantage.

➤ *External desynchronization.* You exit the plane ready for breakfast, but it's dinnertime at your new location. It's dark outside, the traffic is sparse, the shades are drawn across apartment windows, no birds are chirping in the sun, and the daily newspaper won't be delivered for another several hours. You feel disjointed somehow, a little confused and unsettled, and these feelings only progress after you arrive at the hotel and try to sleep when your body urges you to stay awake. This feeling of being out-of-synch with your environment is itself a symptom of jet lag.

➤ *Internal desynchronization.* In addition to feeling "dislocated" because your sense of what time it is differs from the real time in your new location, you also have to cope with a very interesting and little-known side effect of time-zone travel: internal desynchronization, the disruption of your carefully orchestrated biological rhythms. The foremost casualty is, of course, your sleep/wake cycle. Not only may your body be telling you to stay awake during local nighttime, but anxiety, stress, fatigue, and excitement all act together to further disrupt this cycle. Many travelers, for instance, spend less time in the restorative Stages 3 and 4 and REM sleep. They also have more trouble getting to and staying asleep—no matter what time it is locally or internally. In addition, as you may remember from Chapter 2, many of your physiological functions, such as your blood pressure and body temperature, have their own daily rhythms, which are kept in synch by your internal clock. With time-zone travel, all of these rhythms become desynchronized, one from the other, which contributes to your feelings of malaise. Constipation and other symptoms of gastrointestinal distress, headaches, and irritability are just a few of the resulting symptoms. It can take several days for your body rhythms to readjust and run smoothly and in harmony with your new environment.

Night Owl Wisdom

Desynchronization is the disruption of a set pattern of events or processes that normally are coordinated. With jet lag, many different biological functions normally synchronized by the internal body clock become disrupted.

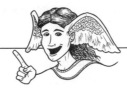

Morpheus Says

Flying north to south—say from Chicago to Rio de Janeiro—is not nearly as disruptive as east-west travel. That's because you don't have to adjust to a vastly different time zone. However, you will suffer from other side effects: fatigue, sleep loss, and symptoms of air travel such as dehydration and irritability. (Later, you'll see that symptoms of jet lag tend to be more severe going east than west as well.)

Go East, Go West

As you may have experienced yourself, the direction of the flight you take significantly influences the degree of jet lag you experience. When you fly eastbound, or against the direction of the sun, jet lag tends to be more severe than when you fly west. That's because when flying westward, you're allowing your body to follow its natural inclination to extend the day to 25 hours. Your bedtime shifts later and later. Let's say you're a New Yorker and you travel to Los Angeles. Within three days, without even trying, your bedtime would quickly shift so that you're going to bed at the same time as your Angeleno counterparts.

By traveling east, on the other hand, you're forcing your body to go against the natural tendency. If you're from San Francisco and travel to Boston, for example, your body will want to keep awake and active (in effect, to extend the day) but, in order to catch up, you'd be best served by going to bed earlier than your body might prefer.

A study of the 1991, 1992, and 1993 records for 19 major-league baseball teams in the Eastern and Pacific time zones of North America shows just how dramatic the difference can be between eastward and westward travel. Those teams that traveled west to east tended to lose the games they played away far more often than those that traveled east to west. The home team won 56 percent of the games, said the researchers, but the probability of winning depended on whether the visiting team had just traveled eastward.

Just for You!

If you're an Owl, you'll probably fare better than Larks when flying west. That's because you naturally want to stay up very late into the night and get up quite late in the day, which helps you advance your sleep/wake patterns. If you're a Lark, eastward travel is better for you, because you find it easier to get up earlier in the morning than to shift to a later bedtime.

Nevertheless, no matter which way you're traveling, for how long, or how far, you're bound to feel some ill effects. You can help minimize those effects in two ways: by preparing well for your journey ahead of time and by working to readjust your biological clock as efficiently as possible.

Be Prepared

Although for most people it's impossible to eliminate all the negative effects of travel on the body and mind, you can help minimize them by being as healthy and well-rested as possible before you get on the plane and by treating yourself well during the flight. Here are a few tips to get you started:

➤ *Get plenty of sleep* before *you travel.* The effects of jet lag are considerably greater if you're already carrying a sleep debt when you travel. Not only will you feel the symptoms of sleep deprivation—excessive daytime sleepiness, headaches, irritability, and so on—but lack of sleep will also exacerbate the disruption of your circadian rhythms.

➤ *Try a gradual approach pre-flight.* If you're traveling west and have some flexibility with your routine, you can try going to bed and getting up an hour later each day for three days before leaving—that way, you'll be on well on your way to meeting the local schedule by the time you arrive. If you're flying eastward, you'll want to reverse the process by going to bed and getting up an hour earlier each day.

➤ *Avoid dehydration.* Airplane travel is highly conducive to dehydration because the air is so dry in the cabin. Dehydration results in diminished blood flow to the muscles, reduced kidney function, and fatigue, all of which exacerbate jet lag. You can prevent dehydration by drinking one liter of water for every six hours of flight time, even if you don't feel thirsty.

➤ *Avoid alcohol.* Alcohol not only affects the quality of your sleep, but also tends to dehydrate the body, two effects you want to avoid if you're trying to alleviate jet lag.

➤ *Exercise.* Although you can't play tennis on board, you certainly can stretch, walk up and down the aisle, and even perform some isometric exercises in your seat. Doing so will help keep your body limber and reduce stress during a long flight.

➤ *Be prepared for sleep on the plane.* In addition to timing your sleep period carefully, you also want to come aboard prepared to improve your sleep environment. Earplugs, an eye mask, an inflatable neck pillow, and a sweater or shawl will help make you more comfortable, and thus more likely to relax and fall asleep.

Wake Up!

Don't wait to grab an airline pillow and blanket. By the time you need to take a nap, more seasoned and adept travelers will have nabbed them all for themselves.

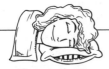

Sleep on it

Use food as medicine. Eating foods high in carbohydrates (bagels, pasta, crackers, etc.) will help boost your levels of serotonin, a brain chemical that acts to relax you and as well as stimulate the release of melatonin, the sleep hormone.

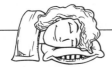

Sleep on it

If you intend to stay less than three days in a new time zone, you can avoid most symptoms of travel-related malaise by simply sticking to your "home" schedule as closely as possible. For example, if you're a Bostonian who flies to London for an afternoon business meeting and only intend to stay one night, time your major sleep period to coincide with Boston rather than London time.

➤ *Eat well.* Generally speaking, it's best to eat several small, light meals throughout the days before, during, and just following your journey. Eating a big, heavy meal will only increase your chances of suffering an upset stomach. Avoid high-sugar snacks, caffeine, and alcohol, all of which can interfere with your ability to sleep and make you feel uncomfortable. Needless to say, airline food is NOT necessarily the best choice for you. We suggest you pack your own healthful "mini-meals" and forgo the on-line service.

Maintaining/Restoring Rhythms

In addition to making it through your journey feeling healthy and vital, you'll also want to speed the rate at which your internal clock adjusts to the time in your new environment. No matter what you do, this process is apt to take at least a couple of days. Of course, the more quickly and well you can fall asleep at local bedtime and wake up feeling rested in the morning, the better. Here are some tips to help you do just that:

➤ *Choose your strategy.* Your very first decision when it comes to your biological clock is whether or not you want to stay on your "home time" or make the adjustment to your new environment. To a large extent, that decision depends on how long you're planning to stay at your travel destination: If it's a very short trip—less than three days—and you have control over your time (you're on vacation, for example), you may be best served by maintaining your home schedule as much as possible. If you're staying longer, or have business meetings to attend that require you to be alert when you'd be sleepy at home, you'll want to readjust your circadian clock as soon as you can.

➤ *Schedule your trip with care.* The best itinerary has you arriving at your destination in the early evening (local time). That way, you'll be able to get a light bite to eat, take a walk to work out the kinks, and have a little time to relax before hitting the sack. Because you'll already be tired from the sheer act of traveling, you may be tired enough to sleep even if it's earlier than usual on "body time." If not, see the information that's coming up on melatonin and light.

➤ *Anticipate your new time zone.* If you're flying when it's nighttime at your destination and it'll be morning when you arrive, try to sleep on the plane. If it's daytime, try to stay awake—no matter what time your body thinks it is at the moment—or at most catch a 20-minute power nap to take the edge off.

➤ *Time your light exposure.* And no, we don't mean for your camera—we mean your body's exposure to light, especially sunlight. Indeed, light therapy can be very helpful in resetting your internal clock, as long as you're careful about when and how long to expose yourself to it. As you may remember from Chapter 11—and we suggest you reread that chapter if you're confused about how light affects your biological clock—exposure to bright light in the morning will help shift you forward, allowing you to go to bed earlier and wake up earlier in the coming days. Bright light in the evening, on the other hand, will shift you back, so that you're going to bed later and getting up later. Combined with taking a dose of melatonin about an hour or so before bedtime, bright-light therapy can significantly speed up your period of adjustment to a new environment.

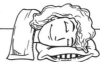

Sleep on it

Some hotels offer extra luxury and pampering for the jet-lag weary: The Bangkok Oriental Hotel, for instance, offers a full spa treatment designed to help "cure" jet lag. It includes hydrotherapy, a papaya body polish, and a massage to unknot cramped muscles. The hotel also offers spa cuisine designed to replace fluids and minerals lost during flight. Whether or not such extras really alleviate the problem, they sure do help you feel better!

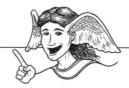

Morpheus Says

Timing light exposure in order to minimize jet lag can be a tricky business, especially if it involves several changes in time zones and destinations over the course of one trip. Circadian Technologies has developed a software program, "Midnight Sun," that combines your itinerary with information about your individual sleep/wake pattern to calculate the dynamic patterns of light and dark, dawn and dusk, and local time throughout your trip. Using this data, the software then creates a prescription for bright-light therapy that will help you reset your biological clock more efficiently.

➤ *Use melatonin wisely.* Taking a dose of melatonin before you want to go to bed at your destination may help set the stage for your body to sleep, even if it's daytime back home. DO NOT take melatonin before this point—if you do, you may end up disturbing your rhythms unnecessarily.

➤ *Avoid using sleeping pills.* Although a quick fix for a travel-related sleep problem may seem like a dream come true (literally!), in the end, you'll probably only make things worse for yourself. The "hangover" effect of most sleeping pills will only increase your feelings of sleep deprivation the next day, and may even make it harder for you to get to sleep the next night.

➤ *Make the most of your hotel.* When you book your hotel, find out what kinds of "jet-lag treatment" services they offer. Some hotels offer rooms equipped with black-out curtains that allow you to sleep even when the sun is shining brightly outside, full-spectrum light sources if you require more light to reset your clock and it's still dark outside, and room service that can prepare whatever meal your body clock desires (dinner at 7 a.m. if need be).

➤ *Nap wisely.* As discussed in Chapter 13, napping can be a godsend when it comes to making up for a sleep loss or preparing the body for a good night's sleep by taking the edge off exhaustion. Once again, though, timing is everything. You'll want to keep your naps short, from 10 to 30 minutes, and avoid napping within 4 to 5 hours of local bedtime.

There's new evidence that the world is getting smaller every day—but your body doesn't necessarily agree! Armed with the advice in this chapter, however, you should be able to improve your chances of having a healthy, happy journey the next time you join the jet set.

Now that you've read about the special kinds of problems—from snoring to parasomnias to narcolepsy to the night shift and jet lag—that can disrupt your sleep, we move on to another topic: How the process of aging from infancy to late life affects your sleep patterns.

The Least You Need to Know

➤ Traveling across time zones can disrupt your body and mind for many different reasons and in many different ways.

➤ Planning your trip wisely and taking care of yourself before and during your journey can help alleviate symptoms.

➤ You can hasten the pace of your internal clock readjustment by wisely using bright light, melatonin, and other techniques.

Part 4
Sleep Through the Life Cycle

Time brings change to almost every aspect of your physical self, and that includes the way you sleep. In the chapters that follow, you'll see how the need for sleep develops from infancy to late life, how sleep patterns change as you age, and the problems that may crop up in different stages of life. We explain some of the reasons these changes occur and offer some suggestions about meeting certain challenges. Then, as an added bonus, we explore something you do throughout your sleeping life: Dream.

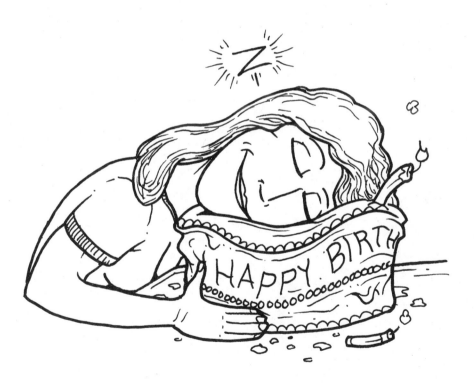

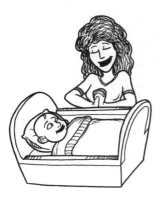

Lullaby and Good Night

Nothing brings more joy—and less sleep—to a family than a new baby. For at least several months, it seems as if you never sleep at all and then, as your baby grows and matures, a host of other bedtime challenges may arise. According to the National Sleep Foundation, about half of all children under six have some kind of sleep problem at some point—and that's to say nothing of the difficulty with sleep experienced by their parents.

The good news is, of course, that most babies and toddlers manage to get all the sleep they need (no matter how disjointed that sleep appears to be to an adult), and that their parents inevitably survive the sleep deprivation triggered by their little bundle of joy. And you will too, especially if you take the time to understand sleep from your child's perspective, a goal we'll help you to meet in this chapter.

Baby Sleep

Although the function of sleep remains a scientific mystery, there are a number of reasons to believe that one role of sleep is related to proper growth and development. And all you have to do is take a look at just how much your new baby sleeps to agree. A newborn sleeps from 16 to 18 hours per day, and it couldn't be just to rest up from her long journey from womb to real life!

Your baby actually started developing her sleep habits in the womb: As early as 22 weeks, she had an alternating pattern of rest and activity, the precursor to BRAC (basic rest-activity cycle) and the adult REM-NREM sleep cycle. This cycle lasts about 40 to 60 minutes, far shorter than the one experienced by the mother, which is 90 to 100 minutes.

What's really interesting is that your new baby is dreaming for about 50 percent of her total sleep time, and even more if she was premature. One can only speculate what a newborn dreams about, but REM sleep (dreaming sleep) appears to be important for the development of certain portions of the brain, specifically the cerebral cortex (the area considered the seat of higher intellectual functions) and the oculomotor system (the area that controls eye movement and sight).

In addition to making up more of a baby's total sleep time, the onset of REM occurs more quickly in infants than in adults. The alteration of NREM and REM sleep, which occurs at approximately 90- to 100-minute intervals in adults, occurs at 50- to 60-minute intervals in infants; in effect, infants have shorter total sleep cycles than adults. Indeed, infants may pass directly from wakefulness to REM sleep, thereby bypassing the first NREM cycle at the beginning of their sleep period.

Just for You!

Although marriage between a Lark and an Owl can be fraught with social and even sexual challenges, it sure comes in handy when it comes to caring for an infant! The Lark can take the early shift without suffering too much, while the Owl's natural tendency to stay up late makes him or her the perfect partner to take the late-night feedings—as long as the Lark mother is not breast-feeding!

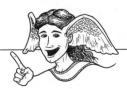

Morpheus Says

Although we'll be using the familiar terms REM and NREM to describe the stages of sleep in your baby and toddler, researchers usually classify the sleep in newborns as either active or quiet. In active sleep, which is the precursor of REM sleep, infants have irregular breathing patterns, move their legs and arms, cry or whimper, and keep their eyes partly open. During quiet sleep, which is NREM in adults, infants have regular breathing and lie very still.

One of the more frustrating challenges for new parents is their baby's unpredictable sleep/wake patterns. Indeed, periods of wakefulness and sleep during the first few months of life can be as short as 20 minutes and as long as six hours. In essence, a baby's adult circadian clock has not yet been set, and the primary Zeitgeber for adults—the rising and setting of the sun—plays little or no role in her sleep/wake patterns. In addition, the pineal gland, which secretes the rhythm-maintaining hormone melatonin, is not yet fully developed in an infant, which helps explain the perfectly normal shorter but less predictable sleep patterns of infancy.

What wakes your baby up is not the sun or another external Zeitgeber but another trigger, primarily a need—for food, a clean diaper, or your attention—that must be met for her to fall back to sleep, no matter what time it is by your clock!

By the time your baby is six months old, however, you should start to get a little respite. At this point, most infants sleep through much of the night; only about 15 percent of infants wake more than once per night. However, don't worry if your baby still has a bit of trouble making it through—the development of sleep patterns is a highly individual matter, and there are no hard and fast rules.

The Crying Game

Your baby suddenly begins to cry loudly and persistently. Her face is flushed, her abdomen tense, and with every cry she draws up her legs as if in terrible pain. She cries and cries—her hands clenched, her feet cold—and still she cries, only stopping when completely exhausted. Your normally angelic little wonder suddenly resembles Satan, and Satan NEVER sleeps. What could be wrong? Sounds like *colic* to us.

Colic usually takes one of two forms. The most common is infantile or "three-month" colic. In this case, your baby will make up for a peaceful day by crying long and hard beginning at nightfall and continuing until well after both you and your baby have passed the level of tolerance. You try burping and patting, diapering and rediapering, cajoling and playing, walking and rocking—and nothing helps. The less common type of colic involves infants who wake every few hours and cry fitfully. These babies may drink small amounts of milk, then fall into a restless sleep.

Night Owl Wisdom

Colic is a condition experienced by infants that causes fussing and crying, often for long periods of the day and night. No one knows what causes colic, or, in fact, what alleviates or cures it. Fortunately, it usually passes on its own by the time a baby is six months old.

What causes colic? The short answer to that question is: No one knows. In some cases, abdominal pain may be the culprit, perhaps caused by an allergy or intolerance to formula or breast milk. Another theory is that children with colic swallow more air than normal, which gets trapped in the intestines and causes pain. Colic may also represent an infant's frustrated reaction to her environment. Since colic usually occurs in the late afternoon and early evening, fatigue may contribute to the severity of a bout. Household activity and tension often increase later in the day, too, as more family members are home, which may add to the baby's distress.

Fortunately, in most cases, symptoms of colic diminish rapidly after a child is three months old and disappear completely by six months.

Sleep Position Counts

Although in what position *you* choose to sleep—on your side, abdomen, back, or tossing and turning—is a largely a matter of preference, the position your baby takes appears to be of critical importance.

About 6,000 to 7,000 apparently healthy babies die every year from a mysterious condition called Sudden Infant Death Syndrome (SIDS). It is a rare event—affecting just two in every 1,000 infants—that occurs in the first year of life, usually between two and four months of age. Researchers believe that SIDS probably has more than one cause. It cannot be predicted, prevented, or reversed.

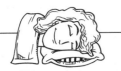

Sleep on it

Make sure to give your baby plenty of "tummy time" while she's awake and you're observing her. She needs to be in that position in order to develop normally. She'll learn to crawl from that position, for instance, which will help her develop strong arm and back muscles.

Since 1992, pediatric sleep experts have been recommending that infants be placed on their backs or sides—as opposed to their tummies—to sleep. The good news is that since that time there has been a 30 percent decrease in SIDS.

Although all parents worry about the health and safety of their infants, it's especially important not to compound the challenge of getting a good night's sleep by needless constant worrying over this rare and unpredictable condition. If there is a history of SIDS in your family, by all means talk to your doctor. Otherwise, place your baby on her side or back, and sleep well.

Settling into a Routine

By about 16 weeks, the total amount of sleep your baby needs drops to about 14 or 15 hours per day. In addition, a clear *diurnal* pattern emerges, meaning that your baby will start to sleep more at night than during the day. Nighttime feedings should start to subside, and weaning your baby from nighttime feedings will help consolidate nighttime sleep. This not only helps you get a good night's sleep but is also important for your baby's sleep development. Don't worry, however, if it takes your baby a while longer before she sleeps through the night (in infants, that translates from about midnight to about 5 a.m.). About one-third of babies still awaken during the night at the end of their first year.

Napping is another important aspect of the sleep of infants and, as we'll discuss further, young children. As an infant ages, the time spent in what we call "naps" during the day also decreases. By six months, nearly 90 percent of all babies take only two naps per day. Early naps, those that occur midmorning, tend to be more active sleep, consisting of more REM and dreaming. Afternoon naps, on the other hand, consist of more quiet or NREM sleep.

By the age of eight months, total daily sleep time is further reduced to about 13 or 14 hours, and a greater and greater percentage of that sleep is quiet NREM sleep. At this point, the transition to sleep shifts from the newborn pattern (wake to active to quiet sleep) to the mature pattern (wake to NREM to REM sleep). By the time a child is about two years old, REM occupies about 20 to 25 percent of her total sleep, an amount that remains relatively constant throughout life.

Night Owl Wisdom

Diurnal is the opposite of "nocturnal," and means both "happening each day" and "occurring in the daytime." Diurnal is sometimes used to describe daily (circadian) rhythms.

In addition to all of the other miracles of development that take place during your baby's first year of life, then, there also occurs these sleep-related changes that signal the healthy development of your baby and—usually—a better, and more regular, sleep/wake cycle for the entire family!

Preschoolers and Sleep

It might seem at first glance that the inconvenience and unpredictability of sleep gives way to a more organized and peaceful situation as your baby grows into her toddler years.

But you're forgetting one thing: As your child matures, she also develops a personality, a will, and a mind of her own. And that's often where the trouble starts when it comes to sleep! Indeed, between the ages of one and two years old, many children start to make a fuss about going to bed. We discuss that at length in the next section. In the meantime, let's see how the sleep/wake patterns continue to mature.

Between the ages of two and five, total sleep time continues to decline slowly, the main sleep period becomes more firmly positioned at night, and daytime sleep needs are usually satisfied by just one short nap. In fact, for most toddlers, a late morning or midafternoon nap means the difference between being a happy camper or a grouchy grinch.

Even if you have trouble getting your toddler to go to bed at night, cutting back on her naps often won't solve the problem. Just as we've pointed out for adults, a missed nap will only make your baby feel overtired and irritable, and thus less likely to sleep restfully. If you find your baby has trouble sleeping through the night, but takes long naps during the day (especially during the late afternoon), talk to your pediatrician about how to manipulate your baby's napping schedule to optimize nighttime sleep.

One of the most remarkable qualities of sleep during toddlerhood is the intensity of the deepest stages of sleep. Most young children begin the sleep period with a rapid descent into Stages 3 and 4 and are usually very difficult to awaken. The intensity of delta sleep may be important for proper growth and development because growth hormones are released during this period.

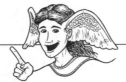

Morpheus Says

In one experiment that shows just how deep a child's sleep can be, children sleeping could not be aroused during Stage 4 sleep even when a loud buzzing sound of 123 decibels—similar to that of a nearby motorcycle—was piped in through the headphones they were wearing. No wonder you sometimes have trouble waking up your toddler!

One of the quintessential aspects of the "terrible twos" (and threes and fours, for that matter) is the bedtime struggle. But even at this young age, establishing a nighttime bedtime ritual is helpful: A bath, diapering, nursing or a bottle, a kiss, a song, and then "into the crib." The importance of this routine is that it establishes a predictable set of events that will help your baby unwind, relax, and get ready for sleep. (But you already know this, having established your own bedtime ritual to help you get to sleep!)

Sleeping Through the Night

Seems like it should be easy, doesn't it? Your baby is working hard all day long at learning and growing, so going to sleep at night should come naturally. But even infants can have trouble getting to sleep, and for a number of reasons.

Among the earliest problems that crop up is the baby's desire to be close to you. Just having you nearby provides comfort and security that helps your baby feel relaxed enough to sleep. Trying to fall asleep away from you can be an upsetting experience, especially as she gets older.

One way to help her cope with her growing independence is with the use of a security blanket, also known as a transitional object. A blanket, stuffed animal, or other easily carried, soft item can become a trusted friend and comforting aid. This object offers your child a bit of extra security at bedtime or in new situations.

Even with a security blanket (and a night light), many infants and toddlers have difficulty going to bed, getting to sleep, and staying asleep and in bed throughout the night. Today, a controversy rages within the pediatric and parent communities between the "Benjamin Spocks" and the "Richard Ferbers." Each of these renowned pediatricians, and their followers, offer a very different approach to getting a child to sleep through the night. The late Dr. Spock advocated a form of tough love that called for parents to put their children to bed at a set time, no matter *how* fussy they are. If they scream and cry, Dr. Spock promoted, let them do so. Do not go into the room or allow the child to leave her bed. Within three nights, the problem will be solved. Or so goes Dr. Spock's theory.

Dr. Richard Ferber, head of the Center for Pediatric Sleep Disorders at Boston's Children's Hospital, offers another, more benign approach. Infants and toddlers, he says, learn by association. Teach them that they can fall asleep only while being held, rocked, or fed, and they'll insist that those conditions be met night after night. If an otherwise healthy child continues to fuss after being put in her crib, Ferber advises parents to give her a reassuring pat and leave the room. If she's still fussy, you can return, reassure her briefly, then leave again. Ferber suggests doing this at increasing intervals—5 minutes at first, then 10, then 15, and so forth. Within a week, she should be fine to fall asleep on her own. (Please note that Ferber offers many variations on this method, and does not advocate this solution for all children.)

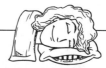

Sleep on it

Don't worry that your child will become too attached to her security blanket. During her normal course of development, she'll eventually lose the need for, and the interest in, this object. You can talk to your pediatrician if you have any concerns, or if you need to help your child make the break with the object as she enters school.

Still other experts think such hard-line approaches are unnecessarily tough on both parents and their children. They feel that the security and comfort of being held while infants fall asleep is an important part of development. In fact, the idea of the "family bed" or co-sleeping has recently come back into vogue. Proponents of the family bed point out that, anthropologically speaking, newborns have always relied on proximity to their mothers to help regulate body heat, breathing, and cardiac rhythms.

Others believe that the disruption to a parent's sleep caused by the kicking and squirming of most toddlers—to say nothing of its effect on marital intimacy—is not worth the potential benefits. Finally, some say that learning to sleep alone allows your child to see herself as an independent individual, and note that it can be difficult to break children of the habit of sleeping with you as they grow older. The decision you make for your family is clearly a highly personal one.

School-Aged Children

As your child grows and develops, she'll establish her own individual sleep personality. She may be a long or short sleeper, needing more or less than the average amount of sleep for her age group; she may have excellent or poor nap-ability, making her a good or not-so-good candidate for daily naps; and she may already show signs of Lark and Owl tendencies.

Generally speaking, the average six- to nine-year-old needs about 10 hours of sleep a night, while the average ten- to twelve-year-old (pre-adolescent) usually sleeps about 7 to 10 hours (and sometimes more, depending on the individual). However, as with younger children—and with adults, for that matter—there are considerable individual variations. In younger children, REM occupies about 26 to 28 percent of the total sleep time, declining to about 15 to 22 percent in the older, pre-adolescent age group. The number of REM periods declines from six per night in the younger group to about four or five in the older group (and in adults).

As school and other social developments occur—the intrusion of television into the evening routine, for example—problems with bedtime may reestablish themselves.

Later in the chapter, we'll discuss some of the ways you can help establish good sleep hygiene habits with your infants, toddlers, and school-aged children. In the meantime, there are some specific sleep disorders you should be aware of that can affect toddlers and school-aged children. Could your child have one?

Sleep Disorders and Your Child

Although most infants and children eventually find their own rhythms and happily make good on the adage "sleep like a baby," others aren't quite so lucky. Among the most common sleep disorders in children are bed-wetting, nightmares and night terrors, bruxism (teeth-grinding), and sleep apnea. Let's take them one by one.

Bed-Wetting

By the time your child is about two or three years old, you'll have worked through the process of toilet training together. Unfortunately it's not at all uncommon for bed-wetting to continue well beyond this. Indeed, about 10 percent of children—from 5 to 7 million children over the age of six—wet their bed.

Although there are almost never any physical long-term effects, bed-wetting often has a psychological impact. A child who wets the bed is apt to feel shame and embarrassment about the problem, as well as anxiety about being accepted by her peers. Bed-wetting often affects school-aged children at a time when the pace of their social development is greatest, as they are beginning to become more independent by sleeping over at friends' homes, going to overnight camps, and so on. A child who wets the bed is likely to avoid such situations out of embarrassment, and thus miss out on some happy milestones. Bed-wetting also can cause sleep disturbances—either the fear of going to sleep and having a bed-wetting accident prevents the child from going to sleep, or wetness and discomfort from an accident wake her up.

Doctors believe that there are many different causes of bed-wetting, including genetic factors. According to *Pediatrics for Parents*, 72 percent of children who wet the bed have one or two parents who also did. In fact, geneticists have located the gene believed to be at least partially responsible for the majority of bed-wetting cases. New research indicates that the absence of a certain hormone—called ADH or anti-diuretic hormone—may cause some affected children to produce as much as four times the normal amount of urine, thus making it difficult for them to hold their bladder through the night.

In some cases, especially in older children with previously good bladder control, bed-wetting enuresis may signal emotional problems such as anxiety and tension. A move to a new house, the arrival of a new baby, or even an exciting upcoming or past event like a birthday party can trigger periods of bed-wetting in some children. Most cases of sporadic bed-wetting can be traced to stress-related triggers.

Only about 5 to 10 percent of all bed-wetting cases have a physical cause, usually a urinary tract infection, diabetes mellitus, or a neurological problem. Sickle cell anemia, kidney failure, lower spine disorders, and premature birth are other potential physical causes. If your child complains of a burning sensation during urination (a sign of a urinary tract infection) or consumes fluids in much greater quantities than usual (a sign of diabetes), make an appointment with her doctor promptly.

In most cases, your child will simply grow out of her bed-wetting problem as she matures. In the meantime, here are some tips to help you with this very common but upsetting problem:

➤ *Reassure your child.* Let your child know that *you* know she isn't wetting the bed on purpose and that you understand how difficult the problem is for her. Another way to offer support and encouragement is to tell your child about another family member who wet the bed but who eventually developed bladder control. This will both give her something to aim for and let her know that the challenge can indeed be met.

➤ *Limit nighttime beverages.* That extra glass of water or juice before bedtime will only exacerbate any problems your child has with holding her bladder. Caffeinated beverages such as cola and iced teas are diuretics, which means that they encourage urination—a double whammy when it comes to sleep problems.

➤ *Avoid shaming or scolding.* Such an approach will only make your child feel more tense and out of control. Remember that your child is not wetting the bed deliberately. Instead, offer her support and let her know how proud you are of her for trying.

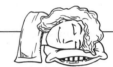

Sleep on it

If your child wets the bed, make the clean-up of accidents as easy as possible. Put a rubber sheet on your child's bed and place a dry towel over the bottom sheet. That way, the mattress will remain free of urine and you can make up a new bed quickly, limiting the amount of sleep both you and your child lose.

Nightmares and Night Terrors

Almost every adult can recall having a nightmare as a child and, indeed, nightmares are very common in children, particularly when they are between the ages of 7 and 10. Scary movies, an anxiety-ridden event (such as getting lost or separated from you)—even an ordinary but highly stimulating day can trigger a nightmare in your child. In most cases, nightmares are no cause for alarm; only if they become chronic and interrupt sleep on a regular basis do you need to mention it to your pediatrician.

The same is true for night terrors, another common childhood phenomenon. Unlike nightmares, which occur during REM sleep, night terrors usually occur in deeper stages of sleep from which a child wakes up suddenly, screaming and highly agitated.

Here are a few ways you can help your child cope if she experiences these generally harmless but always disturbing episodes:

➤ *Understand childhood fears.* The world is a strange, sometimes wonderful and sometimes scary place for toddlers and young children. Each individual child has her own set of fears and worries that may change with each age and stage of development. Talk to your pediatrician or read one of the many excellent books available on childhood development to better understand what might be influencing your child's nightmares and anxiety.

➤ *Keep lines of communication and affection open.* The more you talk to your child and reassure her, the more secure she'll feel, which may help alleviate her nightmares. On the other hand, it's important to understand that even the most well-adjusted, happy child suffers an occasional nightmare or two, and nothing you do, or don't do, can prevent it. Being there when she's frightened, however, may help her get back to sleep more quickly.

Although your child's nightmares are usually no cause for alarm, being there to help her cope and feel secure when she wakes up may help prevent a lifelong problem from developing. A 1996 study in the journal *Sleep* found that lifelong insomniacs took longer to fall asleep and had more fears of the dark and nightmares when they were children than people whose insomnia began in adulthood. They also reported more fears of the dark and nightmares as adults than others. In other words, a child who is afraid of the dark may fret about it and sleep restlessly, an unpleasant experience that in turn escalates the fears. This process can, in some cases, become chronic. If you're there to reassure your child, you may help prevent such a problem from developing.

The Grinding of Teeth

Bruxism, a topic we covered in Chapter 15, is most common in children as their primary teeth begin to grow in and their jaws "search" for a place to rest together. While occasional teeth-grinding is normal and harmless, chronic bruxism can lead to serious dental problems. If you have any questions about your child's experience, talk to your pediatrician or dentist.

Snoring and Sleep Apnea

Although most children snore on occasion, chronic, habitual snoring may be linked to a number of different problems that may warrant medical attention. Enlarged tonsils and adenoids may be obstructing the airway and may require surgical removal. Recent studies also link childhood snoring to Obstructive Sleep Apnea, a potentially serious condition that involves temporary pauses in breathing (see Chapter 14 for more details). Talk to your pediatrician if you have concerns about your child's snoring.

Getting Enough: Your Baby and Your Family

The first few years of your child's life are bound to be thrilling, so you'll want your child and your whole family to be awake and alert enough to enjoy them. Here are some tips to help you all:

➤ *Develop a bedtime routine.* It's never too early to introduce a regular pre-bedtime routine of relaxing activities. The individual elements of the routine will change as your child grows, but the goal is to set the stage for sleep as consistently as possible. Rocking her until she feels drowsy, then singing her a song while she's in her crib every night can help an infant get the idea that it's bedtime. A bath, tooth-brushing, and then reading a story is a good example of a routine that works for a toddler. An older child may want to read to herself before dropping off to sleep. Following your own routine will both set a good example and help you to get ready for bed yourself.

➤ *Set up nap routines as well.* Some children, like some adults, need some help in learning to nap. Eating a light snack, reading a book, then turning out the lights and getting under her blanket may help your child get ready for a nap.

➤ *Create a sleep-friendly environment.* Once again, just like adults, children need a comfortable place conducive to sleep in order to rest well on a regular basis. Make sure your child's room is quiet, dark, and has a comfortable temperature.

➤ *Be a happy, sleep-satisfied parent.* Even if your nap-ability is poor, you'll want to take every opportunity to sleep during the first few months of your baby's life—and that includes taking naps. Although you probably won't be able to avoid becoming at least a little sleep-deprived, napping when your baby naps will help keep you as alert as possible during the day and help you avoid developing uncomfortable side effects, such as headaches and irritability.

The Least You Need to Know

➤ It may take several months for your baby to establish a regular sleep/wake pattern.

➤ Napping remains an important part of toddler's day, helping her to fall asleep at night and remain cheerful during the day.

➤ Sleep disorders can affect infants, toddlers, and school-aged children.

➤ Establishing healthy sleep habits is important at any age.

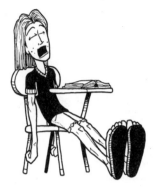

Chapter 20

Teenagers and Sleep

In This Chapter

➤ Exploring the "up-all-night" world of adolescent sleep

➤ Understanding the hormonal connection

➤ Tips for helping your teenager develop good sleep habits

If you're in the process of raising a teenager, you already know that the second decade of life is a period of profound changes of all kinds—social, emotional, and physical. And all of these changes may have an impact on how much—and when—your teenager sleeps. Although sleep problems may seem like the least of your adolescent's challenges, they can, in fact, interfere with his ability to learn, drive, and perform other activities in his busy life.

In this chapter, we'll discuss the importance of sleep in a teenager's life and show you why getting enough sleep may be as difficult for him as it is for you. We'll also suggest some tips that may help improve his sleep now and help him develop good sleep habits for the future.

Why Johnny Can't Get Up

You love him, really you do, but since he hit "that age" he's been a different person from the cooperative, sunshiny little boy you brought up. You can understand his sudden and intense interest in the opposite sex, his reluctance to do the vast amounts of homework he's now assigned, his devotion to afternoon tennis practice. You even understand his extended social life of parties and just hanging out.

But why, you ask yourself, does he need to sleep so late in the day and yet he still seems so tired? He stays up too late, then wonders why he has such a hard time getting up. Just what's going on?

Have you ever wondered why your teenager seems:

➤ More difficult to get up in the morning than a hibernating bear?

➤ Incapable of performing any chore before 11 a.m. on Saturday?

➤ To have become an extreme Owl almost overnight?

➤ Sleepy and distracted at school (according to his teachers) but perfectly alert on weekend afternoons?

It may seem as if he's behaving this way only to annoy you—which may be true, in part, as increasing independence, if not rebellion, is another aspect of the teenage experience. However, there are also some very basic biological factors that may influence his sleep/wake patterns, particularly the hormonal imbalances that occur with *puberty*. They play havoc with all aspects of a teenager's life, including his sleep.

Night Owl Wisdom

Puberty is the time at which the onset of sexual maturity occurs and the reproductive organs become functional. The increase in sex hormone activity stimulates many physical and emotional changes and may affect sleep patterns as well.

Apart from the turmoil caused by the release of large amounts of sex hormones (testosterone for boys and estrogen for girls), other aspects of your child's physiology work against his going to bed and getting up on a regular schedule. In particular, the hormone melatonin, secreted in large amounts during his childhood (accounting in part for the deep sleep experienced by young children), now appears in much lesser quantities. This precipitous drop in melatonin levels may explain the changes in your teenager's sleep/wake patterns.

These changes include:

➤ *Delay in bedtime*. Slowly but steadily, teenagers start to go to bed later and later. At age 10, for instance, most kids go to bed between 9 and 10 p.m., while at age 18, the average bedtime is long after midnight. And on weekends, without the external constraints of school starting times to hold them back, teens tend to go to bed two hours later and wake up about three and a half hours later than they do on school days. In essence, most teenagers, even those who once showed Lark tendencies (and may someday be adult Larks), become Owls for the duration of their adolescence.

➤ *Decrease in total sleep time*. Unfortunately, the delayed bedtime does not result in a correspondingly later wake-up time, especially during high school when school start times prevent teens from sleeping late. The average sleep time declines from about 10 hours before puberty to 8½ hours in mid-adolescence to less than 7 hours in the late teen years. This leaves most teenagers running a steady sleep debt.

➤ *Weekend sleep marathons*. Despite the fact that one of the joys of parenting is the idea that you can get Johnny to clean the garage and mow the lawn on weekends, he's liable to frustrate you by sleeping very late whenever he gets the chance—sometimes well into the afternoon—to try to repay his sleep debt.

Why do these sleep changes occur? A few factors come into play: First, there are the increased demands on a teenager's time. Schoolwork becomes more demanding, involvement in a social life increases, and in many cases, teenagers add a part-time job to their load. Second, hormonal changes make it much more natural for teenagers to want to stay up later and get up later in the morning. In essence, they become at least temporary Owls (some will retain this tendency throughout adulthood) during their high school and college years. And finally, they need more sleep than the average adult because they're still growing and developing. Again, some adolescent sleep experts think that anywhere from 9 to 11 hours of sleep is just about right for most teenagers—far less than what they usually get on most school nights.

In the end, then, your teenager could be just as sleep-deprived—even more—than the average overworked, underpaid, overstressed parent. And this can lead to equally dire results.

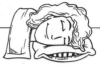

Sleep on it

Letting your teenager sleep late on weekends may be important to his health. Chances are, he's running a sleep debt that sufficient sleep on weekends can help repay. The good news is that he does sleep well once he falls asleep. That is, unless he's suffering from a specific sleep disorder (such as sleep apnea), there's nothing wrong with the quality of his sleep—only the quantity.

The Hazards of Daytime Sleepiness: The Teen Perspective

Dr. Mary Carskadon, a chronobiologist at Brown University of Medicine, Rhode Island, has spent the last 25 years investigating adolescent sleep. According to her studies, the average teenager needs about nine hours of sleep a night to feel rested and stay alert during the day. Unfortunately, according to statistics from her and other studies, most kids only get an average of six hours of sleep during the week at what is a particularly stressful time of life, biologically and socially speaking.

As well as the potential to cause health problems such as increased risk of illness (thanks to a depleted immune system), sleep deprivation affects two particularly significant aspects of a teenager's life: his ability to learn and his proficiency behind the wheel of a car. Let's take them one by one.

Sleep and Learning

In the 1980s, Stanford University was one of the first institutions of higher learning to offer their sleepy students a service once considered the domain of business travelers:

Wake-up calls from operators paid to ring their phones until their clients were at least awake, if not ready to ready to roll. While such a service may seem a luxury, it is clearly a need for students who simply would otherwise be unable to drag themselves out of bed in time for class.

Getting up is just as hard for most American junior and senior high schoolers who have to be at school at around 7:30 a.m. For many, this early start time means that they must get up at 5 a.m. in order to get to school on time—a requirement that goes directly against the natural sleep/wake rhythms of adolescence.

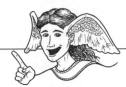

Morpheus Says

A study of 81 private school students performed by Andrew Moore-Ede, Pamela Thacher, and Mary A. Carskadon at Milton Academy in New England showed that virtually all students (99 percent) reported waking before 8 a.m. on school days, while only 19 percent were awake at that time on weekends. On school nights, 43 percent went to bed past midnight, while 73 percent did so on weekend nights. Interestingly, the amount of reported sleep on weekends, 7.8 hours, is still slightly less than the 8 or more hours students felt they needed to feel alert.

Wake Up!

Pulling an "all-nighter" before an exam is likely to backfire. The teen may be able to retain information long enough to answer a few multiple-choice questions, but if the test involves essay questions or other more creative ways of revealing knowledge, chances are his mighty nocturnal effort won't help at all, and may even bring down his grade.

Once out of bed, teens tend to feel tired and out-of-sorts for longer than their pre- and post-adolescent counterparts. At school, then, how much and how well they learn depends a great deal on how much of a sleep debt they're carrying.

Indeed, when adolescents are deprived of one or two nights of sleep, they show marked reductions in alertness and in performance levels on tasks that require attention, memory, cognitive skills, and motor skills.

In a recent study at Johns Hopkins University, published in the February 1998 issue of the *Journal of the American Medical Association*, researchers found that college students got higher grades when they started their first class at 9:30 a.m. instead of 7:30 a.m.

Because of the combination of these social and biological imperatives, a nationwide advocacy movement has begun to move the start time for junior and senior high schools to a later hour. In Edina, Minnesota, for instance, school officials decided to start school at 8:30 a.m. in the fall of 1996, 65 minutes later than the year before. They did so because area physicians lobbied for the new hours, citing studies linking inadequate sleep with lower grades and more frequent car crashes—a subject we cover next.

Sleep and Driving

In Chapters 1 and 12, we discussed the dangers of sleep deprivation on the driving public. Those warnings are especially relevant to teenagers, who are the victims and perpetrators of the highest percentage of traffic accidents by far.

As you may remember from Chapter 1, the U.S. National Highway Traffic Safety Administration estimates that at least 100,000 accidents and 1,500 fatalities per year are due to falling asleep at the wheel—and when it comes to teen drivers, the statistics are even more startling:

➤ Car accidents are the leading cause of death for 15- to 20-year-olds.

➤ Twenty percent of passenger deaths occur when a teenager is behind the wheel, yet teens comprise only 5 percent of the driving population.

➤ Teens are four times more likely to suffer an auto crash than experienced drivers.

➤ Drivers aged 16 and 17 are eighteen times more likely to be killed in traffic accidents than adults aged 30–34.

➤ Five out of 20 teenage drivers will be involved in an auto accident, and more than 1 in 20 teenage drivers will be in an accident that is fatal or results in serious injury.

There are many reasons for the trouble teens have behind the wheel. They include simple inexperience, youthful exuberance, and peer pressure to behave recklessly. In addition, teens are more likely to drive while impaired by alcohol. Indeed, alcohol-related crashes still kill more than 2,000 young people every year, despite the efforts of student and parent groups, such as Students Against Drunk Driving (SADD) and Mothers Against Drunk Driving (MADD), to educate the teen population.

In addition, there's a combination as deadly as teens and alcohol that doesn't get much attention: teens and sleep deprivation. In a study of driving behavior published in a 1996 issue of *Sleep Research*, David Brown, Ph.D., director of the Center for Sleep Evaluation at Optima Health in Manchester, New Hampshire, found that 17 percent of 166 high school drivers reported having fallen asleep at the wheel at least once. Some 64 percent of the students believed that their sleep deprivation worsened their school performance, but only 35 percent felt it impaired their ability to drive.

Yet, according to the National Highway Traffic Safety Administration, half the victims of fatigue-related crashes are under the age of 25. In a North Carolina study, 55 percent of fall-asleep crashes involved people 25 years old or younger, and 78 percent of them were male.

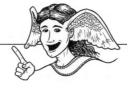

Morpheus Says

In 1989, Michael Doucette, aged 17, won the National Driver's Excellence Contest, earning him the title of "America's Safest Teen Driver." As mentioned earlier, just a few months later, at 5 p.m., Doucette fell asleep at the wheel while driving on a highway near his home in Concord, New Hampshire. The resulting crash killed him and Sharon Link, 19, the driver of another car.

Ironically, in an effort to cut down on drunk driving—but without considering the dangers of driving while sleep-deprived—many communities now encourage all-night, alcohol-free parties, especially at graduation and prom time. Despite the good intentions behind such a plan, the results are often devastating, as it was for a family in Indianapolis who lost their daughter, Amy Lengasher, and her boyfriend, Jason McCaw, both 18, to a fatal car crash. The two had stayed up all night at a post-prom party. McCaw fell asleep at the wheel and was struck head-on by another vehicle when his car crossed the center line. Stories like this one are becoming more and more common across the country.

As you can see, encouraging your teen to get enough sleep—and to recognize the symptoms of sleep deprivation as described in Chapter 1—are essential for his health, safety, and ability to learn and thrive. To a large extent, practicing good sleep hygiene and working to add more hours of sleep to his day will help him feel more rested and more alert. However, you also need to be aware that even teenagers can suffer from a clinical sleep disorder, one that may require medical treatment to solve.

Teens and Sleep Disorders

Although the incidence of some sleep disorders such as sleepwalking, sleeptalking, and bed-wetting tend to diminish during adolescence, and others such as Obstructive Sleep Apnea and insomnia tend to occur more in older adults, adolescents are not immune. The most common sleep disorders in this age group are insomnia and Delayed Sleep Phase Disorder.

➤ *Insomnia.* About 12 to 14 percent of adolescents report frequent insomnia symptoms—and many more report less frequent and very short-term symptoms. The primary symptom is difficulty falling asleep (rather than staying asleep or early awakening, as is true for older adults). They most often attribute this difficulty to feelings of anxiety or worry.

➤ *Delayed Sleep Phase Syndrome (DSPS).* As discussed in Chapter 16, someone with DSPS, if left to her own devices, would go to bed very late at night—often after 3 or 4 a.m.—and get up very late in the morning. While the quality of his sleep would not be diminished, this schedule makes it very difficult for him to meet responsibilities involving school, work, and family. Many adults who suffer from DSPS report having had a childhood or adolescent onset of the symptoms. See Chapter 16 for more information about treating this problem.

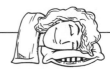

Sleep on it

To test whether your teen suffers from DSPS or just loves to stay up late, see what happens on the weekends. If he's able to get to bed and get up early in order to go skiing or to participate in some other fun activity, chances are he's indulging a natural but controllable preference for late night hours.

Healthy Habits

If there was ever a time in life in which a proper, regular schedule of eating, exercising, and sleep was necessary, adolescence would be it. It's also the time of life when such a schedule is most unlikely.

As a parent of a teenager, you already have your hands full when it comes to setting rules and providing structure. But if your teen is having difficulty with sleep, you might want to see if you can add the following tips to your already full plate of advice:

➤ *Emphasize the need for sleep.* Teenagers already think they're invulnerable to all sorts of challenges and dangers—and not getting enough sleep is probably the last on a long list of things that should have no effect on them. By all means, show your teen this chapter, especially the information about the potentially deadly effects of drowsy driving.

➤ *Set limits.* Although your teen may have a biological preference for a later schedule, it's not imperative that he indulge it. With a little structure and some regularity, he can shift his clock to a more reasonable time. If he's gotten into the habit of staying up until 1 or 2 a.m., insist that he go to bed 30 minutes earlier each of the next several nights until he can enjoy at least $7^1/_2$ to 9 hours of sleep each night.

➤ *Establish a bedtime routine.* Turning off the television, computer, and telephone at least an hour before your teen's bedtime will give him some time to quiet his mind before trying to sleep. Structure of any kind may seem anathema to the very idea of being a teenager, but it's worth a shot.

➤ *Make the stress-exhaustion connection.* Most teenagers find themselves under pressure on many fronts—school, social life, dating, parental expectations—that can overwhelm them. Although it's highly unlikely that your teen will jump at the chance to meditate or practice other forms of stress reduction, just getting him to talk about the pressure he faces might help.

➤ *Watch caffeine intake.* Caffeine is the most readily accessible stimulant in the country—and teens are just as likely to use and abuse it as adults. Remember, caffeine isn't found only in coffee, but also in soft drinks, chocolate, and other foods. See if you can get your teen to lay off the caffeine after 6 p.m. It might just help him turn in earlier in the evening.

➤ *Encourage exercise.* It's never too early to make exercise a regular part of daily life. Exercise helps reduce stress and keep the body fit, which can certainly make it easier for young and old alike to get better sleep. If your teen isn't involved in organized sports, encourage him to participate in more solitary activities like bicycling, jogging, or walking.

➤ *Suggest napping as an approach.* At first, it may seem absolute anathema to your teenager to take an afternoon nap, but it may be the best way for him to catch up on sleep. If he times it well—say between getting home from school and dinnertime—a nap can not only help him get to sleep more easily at bedtime, but also to study after dinner.

➤ *Offer this book.* Throughout Part 2, we offered hundreds of tips for sleeping well that may help your teen as well as you sleep better. If he's really having trouble with daytime sleepiness, he may benefit from learning about good sleep hygiene habits such as those covered in Part 2.

Now that you've read about the sleep habits of babies and teenagers, it's time to move forward—to the challenges of young adulthood and middle age. Although often less fraught with sleep disorders and difficulties than other stages of life, the middle years have their own set of sleep-related challenges, as you'll see in the next chapter.

The Least You Need to Know

➤ Sleep problems are common in teenagers.

➤ Sleep deprivation makes learning more difficult at a crucial time in a person's life.

➤ Drowsy driving is just as dangerous—perhaps even more dangerous—in a teenager than in an adult.

➤ Adolescence is the perfect time to begin to develop proper sleep habits.

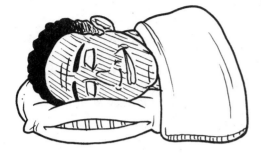

Chapter 21

Through the Middle Years

In This Chapter

➤ Understanding sleep through the middle years

➤ Exploring the connection between psychological stresses and sleep difficulties

➤ Focusing on the special sleep problems faced by women

➤ Learning to make adjustments as you age

In previous chapters, we've discussed the most common sleep problems and solutions, ranging from insomnia caused by stress and poor sleep hygiene to sleep disorders like apnea and the parasomnias. For those of you in the middle stage of life—say from your mid-20s to your mid-40s—you'll find most of what you need to know about sleep and sleep solutions in those chapters. That's also true for those of you in this age group working the night shift or struggling with the effects of time-zone travel.

In this chapter, we discuss three primary issues: First, your sleep patterns—which have remained relatively stable during your 20s and 30s—may begin to change as you enter your mid-40s. It is therefore important for you to re-evaluate your needs at this time. Second, we discuss the disruptions to a "normal" sleep pattern that can emerge with a psychological problem like depression or anxiety, which is very common in the middle years.

We then focus on one group of adults particularly vulnerable to sleep problems: women. That's right. Virtually half our population is faced with special sleep-related challenges, thanks in large part to the wonderful world of hormones. But we'll get to that later. In the meantime, here's what the next stage of life looks like in terms of your natural sleep/wake patterns and just what might interfere with them.

Establishing Your Adult Pattern: An Evaluation

You've made it through infancy, when what woke you up had more to do with your feeding schedule than your biological clock. Toddlerhood was no picnic, either, thanks to the nightmares and insecurity issues you had to face. Sleep wasn't such a bad thing when you were around seven or eight, when it seemed like you could sleep through anything, but adolescence was tough—for lots of reasons, of course, but also because your sleep/wake patterns just didn't fit into the outside world's idea of a 24-hour day.

Fortunately for most people, in the decades between adolescence and later life (from your mid-20s to about your mid-40s), sleep itself becomes more routine. Your true Sleep Personality shines through, and with luck, you'll learn to make the most of it. If you're a Lark, you might use those early morning hours to exercise or get household chores out of the way before heading to work. Owls, on the other hand, especially those of you who thrive into the late hours of the night, might find yourselves drawn to shift work or freelance situations in which night work is welcome. Long sleepers figure out a way to make a 9- or 10-hour sleepfest fit into most days, while dedicated nappers become adept at shutting out the world in the middle of the day.

That's in the best of all possible worlds, of course. If you're reading this book, however, and aren't suffering from a either a short-term psychological upset or a chronic sleep disorder, it's clear that something about your natural sleep patterns and the real world you live in just aren't meshing.

Take another look at Chapter 5. Did you really take the time to evaluate your Sleep Personality, and did you really take what you learned to heart? Or are you still caught up with the idea that everyone should get 8 hours of sleep a night, or that sleep is just a waste of time? If you are, we hope you'll take the time to rethink your approach to sleep, especially as it relates to your own particular challenges, problems, and natural tendencies. This is especially important as you get older, particularly as you enter your early 40s, because that's when things often begin to change.

Indeed, if there ever were a crucial time to re-examine your sleep habits, it's as you enter your 40s. At this stage of life you're liable to experience some subtle—or not so subtle—changes to your Sleep Personality, changes that are likely to become even more marked the older you get. For instance, many people find that they're far less flexible about sleep, less able to adapt to changes in their schedules, than they were when they were younger. Symptoms of sleep deprivation may occur sooner and affect you more profoundly. Jet lag may be more difficult to manage, and you may find yourself less able to tolerate the effects of alcohol or caffeine. And sleep disorders, particularly Obstructive Sleep Apnea, may first appear as you enter middle age.

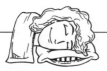

Sleep on it

If you're entering your early 40s and haven't filled out your Sleep Log recently, now is the time to do it. You're bound to learn a lot about how well (or poorly) you sleep, as well as how your sleep habits and preferences may be changing. By keeping track of your sleep patterns, you might be able to identify more helpful solutions to any sleep problems that crop up.

No one really knows why such problems start emerging (or re-emerging) at this stage of life. In Chapter 22, we discuss some of the current theories, including one that focuses on a weakening of the biological clock that occurs as a side-effect of the aging process. We do know for sure, however, that such changes commonly occur at this time, which means you should pay special attention to your own sleep patterns as you pass through your 40s. The more you know about them and how they change, the better prepared you'll be for the challenges you may face in late life.

In the meantime, we thought it might be helpful to discuss the impact of psychological problems, specifically anxiety and depression, on your sleep patterns. Although these conditions can and do affect people of all ages, they are most common in men and women in the middle decades of life.

Psychology and Sleep

As the *Encyclopedia of Sleep and Dreaming* succinctly puts it, "Troubled minds have troubled sleep." Back in Chapter 8, we discussed stress, that nebulous but relevant term used to describe any external pressure that affects your health and well-being in general, and your sleep patterns in particular. As discussed, stress can affect you at any stage of life, which is why we devoted a whole chapter to understanding what causes it and what it can do to the body and mind.

In addition to "ordinary" stress, there are two relatively common psychological disorders that have a direct impact on sleep: anxiety and depression. Let's take a look at each one.

Sleep Robber #1: Anxiety

Anxiety is a broad term used to describe an intense fear or dread. In some cases, you know just what's causing your feelings: It could be an upcoming event, financial problems, or the illness of a loved one. In other cases, anxiety lacks a clearly defined cause but rather involves a kind of uneasiness or distress about life's uncertainties.

According to the National Comorbidity Study, as many as one in four men and women in the United States may experience an *anxiety disorder* at some point in their lives. In fact, more than one-third of all individuals who consult mental health professionals do so because of an anxiety disorder.

There are several types of anxiety disorders. Some involve episodes of sudden, inexplicable terror

Night Owl Wisdom

Anxiety disorders are a group of mental illnesses that involve feelings of unease and fear that interfere with one's ability to perform normal, day-to-day activities. They cause both physical and psychological symptoms.

(panic attacks); others, inordinate fears of certain objects or situations (phobias); and still others, chronic distress (generalized anxiety disorder). All of these conditions can upset your ability to sleep.

As you may remember from Chapter 8, feelings of anxiety and stress trigger the "fight-or-flight" response, in effect readying the body for action not sleep. Indeed, the biochemical components of this response—the chemicals released that stimulate the body—may have a direct influence on the brain's sleep mechanisms.

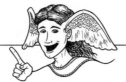

Morpheus Says

Post-traumatic stress disorder, the overwhelming feelings of anxiety and stress that occur after a physical or emotional trauma, may trigger extremely disturbing nightmares that relive the event. Called post-traumatic nightmares, they are accepted as one of the diagnostic symptoms of post-traumatic stress disorder.

Symptoms of an anxiety disorder include the following:

➤ Episodes of overwhelming fear, rapid heartbeat, chest pain, profuse sweating, trembling, and shaking

➤ Avoidance of certain things, places, or situations because of anxiety

➤ Persistent feelings of anxiety, apprehension, restlessness, or irritability

➤ Difficulty with concentration

➤ Difficulty in falling or staying asleep

The more of these symptoms you experience, the more reason you have to be concerned about anxiety disorders, especially if they have persisted for more than a month or are interfering with your work or social life. It's very important to seek medical treatment for your problem—it's not something that's likely to go away on its own, especially if it's already been troubling you for some time. Fortunately, successful treatment, ranging from medication to talk therapy to stress reduction techniques, can help alleviate anxiety, which almost always automatically leads to a better night's sleep.

Anxiety often occurs together with another sleep robber—depression. More than just "the blues," depression is a serious medical disorder that can undermine your general health and play havoc with your natural sleep/wake patterns.

Sleep Robber #2: Depression

After anxiety disorders, depression is the most common mental health disorder in America today, affecting close to 20 percent of the population. The most common age group for depression is between 20 and 44. About one in four women and one in ten men will develop depression during this period.

Depression is a medical disease that appears to be caused by an imbalance of brain chemicals responsible for transmitting messages about mood and behavior. When these chemicals no longer function efficiently, a number of symptoms may result. They include:

➤ *Emotional disturbances*, such as crying, hopelessness, guilt, and despair

➤ *Behavioral changes*, such as social withdrawal, loss of interest in activities, and increase in alcohol use or abuse

➤ *Somatic complaints*, including pain, headaches, decreased energy, gastrointestinal distress, appetite changes, loss of sex drive, and sleep problems (either insomnia or hypersomnia [excessive sleeping] that interferes with daily activities)

Wake Up!

Problems with sleep can be caused, or complicated, by psychological problems such as anxiety, depression, and drug and alcohol abuse. That's why it's important to see your doctor on a regular basis, and to discuss with him or her ALL of your symptoms, including sleep difficulties, use or abuse of drugs or alcohol, and mood changes.

Chronic insomnia is linked not only to daytime sleepiness and other problems but also to depression and other psychological conditions. A National Institute of Mental Health study found that people who said they had insomnia had a higher risk of later developing a major depressive disorder than those who had slept adequately. More than half the insomniacs studied worldwide by the World Health Organization had problems with anxiety, depression, or alcohol abuse.

Sleep problems are, in fact, one of the hallmark symptoms of depression. Patients with depression complain often of fragmented sleep, with difficulty falling asleep and frequent middle-of-the night awakenings. Another common sleep disturbance in depression is early morning awakening, sometimes as early as 3 a.m., and the inability to fall back asleep. That could be why F. Scott Fitzgerald, who suffered from bouts of depression himself, once wrote, "In a real dark night of the soul, it is always three o'clock in the morning." Although morning awakenings tend to be the most common symptom of this chemical imbalance, some people with depression may sleep too much.

Why are sleep problems so common in depression? Research suggests that the connection may be a deep one. One theory suggests that depression may be caused in part by an imbalance between serotonin, a brain chemical known to promote sleep and elevate mood, and *acetylcholine,* a chemical known to cause sleep disturbances. Another theory centers on a disruption of circadian rhythms as the cause of depression.

The connection between mood and sleep has led some researchers and clinicians to explore sleep deprivation as a treatment for depression. One night of total sleep deprivation, sleep deprivation in the second half of the night, or selectively depriving a patient of REM sleep have all been shown to improve symptoms in depressed patients, although once the patient catches up on sleep, the symptoms often re-appear. Nevertheless, such positive outcomes may result because sleep deprivation somehow helps to rebalance neurotransmitters and hormones involved in both sleep and depression.

Diagnosing depression—differentiating it from other medical illnesses as well as separating it from normal dips in mood and energy—is a job best left to professionals, as is treating it. In fact, the diagnostic criteria set forth by the American Psychiatric Association are quite specific. If you suffer from more than a few of the symptoms we listed earlier, we suggest you see your doctor soon for an evaluation. More than 80 percent of all people with depression can be successfully treated with medication, psychotherapy, or a combination of the two.

Women and Sleep

When it comes to sleep, it appears that women in general are more vulnerable to insomnia and other problems than their male counterparts.

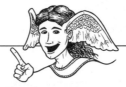

There are two main reasons for the exhaustion experienced by so many women. First, today's generation of women enjoy less leisure time than almost any generation before them. According to the National Commission on Sleep Disorders Research, the average American has added 158 hours per year to his work schedule since 1969. For working mothers, the increase has been a whopping 241 hours.

The other reason is biological. The fluctuating hormones involved in the menstrual cycle, and the changes that occur with pregnancy and then menopause, frequently affect sleep as well.

Your Cycle and Sleep

Surprisingly few studies address the effect of the menstrual cycle on sleep, and those that do show inconsistent results. However, many women notice changes in their sleep patterns during their monthly cycle.

Some studies implicate the rise and fall of *progesterone*, the female hormone that prepares the womb for pregnancy during the second half of the cycle, in the sleep changes in women. Here's how it might work:

➤ Low progesterone levels during the beginning of the menstrual cycle may interfere with deep sleep, leaving women feeling a little sleep deprived even if they've slept their normal number of hours.

➤ When ovulation starts, *progesterone* levels rise, which can cause an improvement in sleep quality and an increase in sleep quantity.

➤ As menstruation begins, levels of both progesterone and estrogen drop, potentially making sleep more difficult to obtain.

Again, studies proving the connection are sparse and inconclusive, and many women find their sleep patterns do not coincide with this theory. For instance, many women find themselves feeling especially sleepy during menstruation and have more difficulty with sleep at the beginning of their cycles. Keeping a diary can help you determine when in your cycle you should make an extra effort to avoid caffeine, late afternoon or evening workouts, and other factors that exacerbate the problem.

Night Owl Wisdom

Progesterone is the female sex hormone released during the second half of the menstrual cycle that helps prepare the womb for pregnancy.

Those Special Nine Months

Many women report daytime sleepiness during the first trimester of their pregnancy, possibly caused by an increase in the hormone progesterone, which is known to have a sedative effect. One way to combat fatigue is to try to fit in a quick nap at lunchtime whenever possible; eating small snacks frequently throughout the day also seems to help. By the second trimester, most women find that they have as much energy as they had before becoming pregnant, sometimes more. During the third trimester, women are generally tired enough, and willing enough, to sleep and sleep well, but they may have difficulty sleeping because they simply can't get comfortable.

Change of Life, Change of Pattern

One of the harbingers of menopause is hot flashes—feeling hot and flushed—caused by a widening of blood vessels near the skin's surfaces brought on by fluctuating levels of estrogen. Not surprisingly, these variations in body temperature can have a substantial impact on restful sleep.

In addition to the symptoms of menopause affecting sleep, estrogen levels appear to be a factor. Before menopause, estrogen seems to protect women from apnea, but as hormonal levels decrease, snoring and sleep apnea can become common.

Learning to Make Adjustments

Throughout this book, we've offered you all kinds of advice about getting better sleep under all kinds of circumstances. What we hope you've come away with, most of all, is that the way you sleep is every bit as unique to you as your personality or the color of your eyes. Understanding your natural style, and learning to adapt it to the stresses and strains of everyday life, will help you sleep better today and tomorrow.

Indeed, you're getting older every day and, sooner or later, you'll be heading into late life, a time of many changes including some that involve your sleep patterns. That's a subject we'll discuss in the next chapter.

The Least You Need to Know

➤ Your natural sleep personality emerges in full force during the middle decades of your life, but may begin to change as you enter your mid-40s.

➤ Anxiety and depression, the two most common psychological disorders of mid-life, both have sleep problems as major symptoms.

➤ Women have special sleep problems throughout their lives due to the fluctuating nature of female hormones.

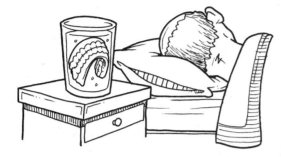

Chapter 22

Sleep Challenges of Late Life

According to a 1998 National Sleep Foundation survey, 42 percent of American adults believe that the older you get, the fewer hours of sleep you need. Unfortunately, nothing could be further from the truth. Although sleep patterns change significantly as you age—and we'll show you how and why in this chapter—your need for sleep remains fairly constant. Indeed, adequate sleep is an essential part of physical and emotional health at every stage of life, perhaps especially as the aging process begins to take its toll on the body.

In this chapter, we'll discuss some of the most common sleep challenges related to aging and provide some tips on getting better sleep in your later years.

Sleep and Aging: The Challenges

Aging: We all do it. It's an inevitable part of the life cycle, and so far, in spite of the mighty efforts made in laboratories around the world, no magical or medical cure for it has yet been discovered.

The skin wrinkles, muscles weaken, hair turns gray, and, eventually, body systems just aren't as efficient as they once were. Look around you and you'll see what we mean. More and more Americans are entering their golden years every day. Ponder this statistic: In 1980, there were 26 million Americans age 65 and older; in 2030, that number will swell to over 70 million. And imagine this: Every seven seconds another *baby boomer* turns 50 in the United States today.

Night Owl Wisdom

A **baby boomer** is a man or woman born in the United States between 1946 and 1964, a time of one of the greatest surges in birth rates in this country. Today there are about 78 million baby boomers, representing 30 percent of the population.

But why, you ask, must we grow old? Well, that's a question without a definitive answer. But here's one reason: We age and finally die in order to make room on this planet for the next generation of human beings to live and thrive. Should the mortality dramatically fall—if fewer people got old and died than were born—the earth could become pathologically overpopulated, which would strain natural resources and thus put the entire ecosystem in jeopardy.

On the molecular level, the same general theory holds true. In a young and healthy body, new cells replace those that die in an orderly fashion. But as we age, cells within the body are neither repaired nor replaced. Eventually, the system or organ affected by cell death or mutation will no longer function properly. And, because human physiology is so interdependent, disruption in one part of the body often has widespread effects.

The first overt sign that the process has begun occurs to the skin. Wrinkles develop in part because the body no longer replaces the cells that make up the top layer of skin (the epidermis) as often. Collagen, a protein that forms 97 percent of the middle layer of skin (the dermis), starts to die at a greater rate than it is reproduced. Thus the skin loses some of its elasticity and density and develops wrinkles as the tissue begins to fold in upon itself.

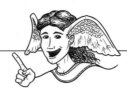

Morpheus Says

Does how much, or how little, you sleep affect how long you live? That's a question without a definitive answer as yet. But a 1959–1960 study of about one million adult men showed that subjects who said that they usually slept either much less than 6 hours or much more than 9 hours were more likely to die at a faster rate than those who slept closer to the average of 7 to 8 hours per night. (See the following "Sleep and Mortality" figure.) Up to now, research has not explained why long and short sleep are associated with early death—and there may be many other as yet unknown factors involved.

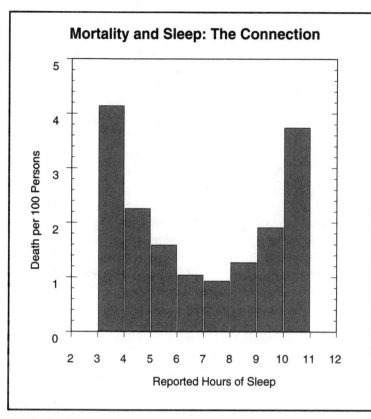

Mortality and Sleep: The Connection

How much you sleep on the average may have an effect on how long you live. A study of over a million adult men showed that people who sleep very little (less than 4 hours per night) or quite a lot (more than 10 hours per night) tend to die at a much faster rate than someone who sleeps in the middle range, from 5 to 9 hours of sleep on average. However, the graph does not prove cause and effect. It might be that the very sickest people either sleep poorly or sleep excessively.

From Kripke, D et al, Arch. Gen. Psychiatry 36, 1979, with permission.

Another sign of aging is the graying of your hair, which occurs in a similar manner: Hair turns gray because the body produces less and less pigment—the substance that gives hair its color—the older we get. Although a tendency for early graying is hereditary, everyone eventually turns gray: By the age of 50, more than half the population has gray hair and the percentage continues to grow with each decade of life. Inch by inch, body part by body part, organ by organ, age-related changes take place, moment by moment, year after year. Some changes are subtle, some dramatic, some reversible, some not. But you've got to live with them, one way or another. And it's better than the alternative, right?

The good news is that we're living longer, and generally better, than ever before. Advances in medicine and in the social structure of the country are making it possible to live a full and vital life far past the standard age of retirement. In fact, did you know that more than half of all people over the age of 85 live independently at home? That makes it more important than ever that you learn how to spend those years AWAKE and alert! Your body, however, may have other ideas.

Changing Sleep Patterns

As if the wrinkles and gray hair weren't enough, however, you'll also find that your sleep patterns begin to change as you get older. As mentioned in Chapter 21, as you enter your mid-40s, you're likely to find that sleep—the process and timing of it—just isn't the same as it was in your younger days. You might discover that jet lag affects you more now, that staying asleep through the night is becoming the exception rather than the rule, and that you're in bed before the 11 o'clock news and awake to see the sunrise more often. In other words, you'll slowly but surely become more of a Lark and less of an Owl, no matter what Sleep Personality you had in your youth. And those changes only intensify the older you get.

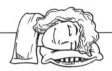

Sleep on it

Although you should expect to start to wake up and go to bed earlier as you get older, be aware that extreme changes in your sleep habits may indicate a sleep problem called Advanced Sleep Phase Syndrome (ASPS) that may require some professional help to handle. See Chapter 16 for more information.

Not only does *when* you sleep change, *how* you sleep does too. As you age, you spend less and less time in deep Stages 3 and 4 sleep and more in the lighter Stages 1 and 2. You're also less efficient at sleep: You may have trouble getting to sleep or staying asleep, and you may wake up too early. In young adults without sleep problems, over 95 percent of the time spent in bed may be spent asleep. By the age of 65, a sleep efficiency of 80 percent or even lower is quite common.

Unfortunately, your need for sleep does not diminish along with your ability to sleep. Some studies with the Multiple Sleep Latency Test (you remember: the test we described in Chapter 4 that measures how sleepy you are by observing how long it takes you to fall asleep during your normal waking hours) have shown that older adults tend to be more physiologically sleepy than younger people during the day. Most older people also take more time to respond to light, sound, and touch, another sign that the elderly simply aren't as alert as their younger counterparts.

What Goes Wrong

Why would sleep patterns break down with age? That's a question that sleep researchers continue to ponder. It seems likely that aging involves a gradual weakening of the biological clock, which disrupts a host of crucial cycles throughout the body. Such a weakening could be both a cause and a symptom of the aging process. In other words, your internal clock is probably just as vulnerable to cell breakdown and degeneration as your hair, skin, and organs. The disruption in cycles—of blood pressure, hormone secretion, and so on—may result in the diseases and degeneration related to aging as well as in the changes to your sleep patterns.

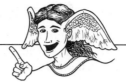

Morpheus Says

A 1998 study, presented at the annual meeting of the Society for Neuroscience, showed that people in different age groups estimate time differently—and that the ability to estimate time declines with age. When asked to estimate when three minutes had passed, people in their early 20s were accurate within three seconds, while people in their 60s estimated that three minutes were up after three minutes and 40 seconds had passed. Middle-aged subjects fell in between but, like the older people, all underestimated the passage of time. The problem could be a decline in dopamine, a neurotransmitter that appears to speed up this internal clock.

We do know that far more than biology is involved, both in what makes us "old" and in the changes that occur to our sleep patterns as we age. A variety of physical, emotional, and lifestyle factors also have a great deal of influence on how much, how well, and how long we sleep.

Lifestyle Issues

Assuming you developed healthy eating and exercise habits during your youth and middle age, if you're like many older Americans, more and more of those habits go by the wayside as each year passes. You tend to get less exercise and pay less attention to eating a balanced and nutritious diet than you did in your younger days—and that's all the more true if you live in a nursing home or assisted living situation. As we've discussed, men and women of any age who get regular exercise report better sleep, and those who remain at a healthy weight do the same.

Another sad truth about many people as they get older, particularly after they retire from the workplace, is that they tend to live more isolated and unstructured lives. Not only does this sense of isolation have profound psychological effects, it may also affect the ability of their biological clocks to keep proper time. Remember, the sun isn't the only Zeitgeber we have: Eating meals and exercising at regular times, catching the same evening train home, performing chores every Saturday—all of these activities help to maintain the psychological and biological rhythms of life.

Illness and Other Physical Factors

We hate to bring up a sore subject, but aging inevitably brings illness. Some of us stay healthy a lot longer than others, partly because we lead healthier lives and partly because of the sheer luck of the genetic draw. In the end, though, we're all vulnerable.

As we discussed in Chapter 4, any number of illnesses—and the medications that treat them—can cause sleep disturbances, and many of those diseases, including heart disease, chronic respiratory conditions, and neurological disorders like Parkinson's disease, are more likely to occur later in life. Any condition that causes pain, particularly arthritis, can also disrupt sleep in your later years.

There are three specific conditions that directly affect sleep and occur almost exclusively in an older population: One is Alzheimer's disease (and other forms of dementia), another is nocturnal urination, and the other is menopause. Let's take a brief look at how each problem can disrupt sleep:

➤ *Alzheimer's disease and other dementias.* Although losing mental capacity is perhaps the greatest fear associated with aging, the vast majority of people age through their 60s, 70s, and even 80s without suffering any serious decline in their ability to remember or learn new facts. That said, about 15 percent of older people eventually do develop *dementia*, an organic brain disorder that interferes with mental function and that tends to grow worse with time. The incidence increases with age; about 50 percent of people over age 85 suffer some symptoms of dementia, and approximately 60 percent of these individuals suffer from the type of dementia called Alzheimer's disease (AD).

One of the most common symptoms of AD and other dementias are sleep problems. People with dementia have trouble getting and staying asleep, and they spend most of their time in light Stages 1 and 2 sleep. In some cases, they also have a reduction in the amount of time they spend in REM sleep. Needless to say, these individuals tend to be in a constant state of sleep deprivation in addition to suffering other symptoms.

Approximately 30 percent of those with dementia also experience sundowner's syndrome. They become agitated and restless—even aggressive—in the late afternoon or evening. Some doctors think that sundowning may be related to a sleep disorder caused by a disruption in normal body rhythms. In fact, there is some evidence that sundowning may be more common in the winter months, with their earlier and longer periods of darkness and subdued lighting, which links it to Seasonal Affective Disorder. Sundowning's possible relationship to the sleep disturbances of dementia suggests that it may reflect a more generalized dysfunction of circadian rhythms.

Currently, no cure for Alzheimer's disease or other dementias exists, and treatments are few and far between. In these cases, doctors usually prescribe sleeping pills to help sufferers get the sleep they need.

➤ *Noctural urination.* As the aging process continues, more and more men develop problems with nighttime urination, a condition called *nocturia*. In many cases, a disorder of the prostate gland is responsible. A gland located within the pelvis, beneath the bladder, the prostate surrounds the urethra, the duct through which urine passes. This gland plays an important function in reproduction by contributing fluids to the semen.

As men age, it is common for the prostate gland to enlarge and thus interfere with urination. This condition is also known as *benign prostatic hypertrophy.* The National Institute of Health reports that more than four out of every five men between the ages of 50 and 60 have benign enlargement of the prostate gland. Cancer of the prostate is less common, but ranks third among the types of cancer that kill American men. It is most frequent in men aged 60 to 80.

In most cases, an enlarged prostate gland is not serious and often requires no treatment. However, if the symptoms are severe, the condition can be corrected surgically. With regular check-ups and testing, prostate cancer can be detected early, in which case it can almost always be cured.

➤ *Menopause.* As discussed in Chapter 21, menopause-associated hot flashes are one of the prime causes of sleep deprivation in women. Sleep laboratory studies show that nearly every hot flash during sleep prompts an arousal, and that women with hot flashes sleep less efficiently than those without them, waking up more often and staying awake longer. Even women who do not suffer hot flashes experience more fragile sleep following menopause.

Night Owl Wisdom

Sundowner's syndrome is a term used to describe periods of nocturnal confusion and agitation that usually occur in the late afternoons to elderly people who suffer from **dementia**, an organic brain disease that causes loss of memory and other cognitive and behavioral changes.

Night Owl Wisdom

Benign prostatic hypertrophy is a common condition in men over the age of 50 involving the enlargement of the prostate gland. This condition can lead to difficulties with urination, including **nocturia**, the urgent need to urinate during the night that results in sleep problems.

Estrogen replacement therapy (ERT) has been shown to alleviate the symptoms of menopause, including the hot flashes that so often wake up women at this stage of life. ERT is not without risk, however, and you should discuss the matter with your physician at the appropriate time.

Psychological Factors

Although more and more people find late life to be a time of opportunity and freedom to explore new horizons, this freedom usually does not come without a price. Worries and anxieties about the future, the loss of your sense of self after retirement, and the grieving over the deaths of loved ones are just a few of the challenges we face as we get older. As we discussed in depth in Chapter 8, stress of any kind can certainly have a negative effect on your ability to sleep, which may help explain why so many older people struggle with this problem.

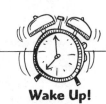

Wake Up!

When you're traveling, be aware that as you age, your ability to tolerate time-zone travel may decrease. Many older people have more trouble with jet lag than they did in their younger days. For reasons not yet well understood, this tends to affect older men—who appear to have more problems sleeping at new times than younger men and women of any age.

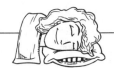

Sleep on it

If you or a loved one lives in a nursing home or is bed-bound, it's important to create a distinct sense of day and night even inside. That means bringing light into the room as much as possible during the day, and making the room as dark and quiet as possible at night.

Some Solutions

So far, of course, there's no cure for aging. You can, however, limit the "symptoms" associated with the process for as long as possible by living a healthy life: eating well, exercising regularly, and staying connected to friends, family, and your own interests as much as possible.

Here are a few tips that may help you or someone you love make sleep in late life a satisfying, restorative activity:

➤ *Practice proper sleep hygiene.* The best advice we can give you is to reread the chapters in Part 2 and do your best to improve your sleep habits. That means cutting back on caffeine, avoiding alcohol, exercising regularly, reducing stress, creating an environment conducive to sleep, and getting out into the sun every day.

➤ *Limit time in bed.* People hoping to make up for lost sleep often go to bed earlier and stay in bed longer, further disrupting their sleep patterns. If you're otherwise healthy, limit your time in bed to no more than 9 hours total—including naps—within a 24-hour period.

➤ *Get outside.* Thirty or more minutes of regular daylight exposure is the best stabilizer of circadian rhythms. If you find yourself waking up too early in the morning, you'll benefit most by getting late evening exposure to artificial light with an intensity of 2,500 to 10,000 lux. (See Chapter 11 for more information.)

➤ *Exercise.* It's true at any age: Regular exercise means better general health and, on average, better sleep. In a study reported in a 1997 issue of *Journal of the American Medical Association*, those people aged 50 to 76 years who engaged in low-impact aerobics and brisk walking for 30 to 40 minutes four times a week for 16 weeks gained about an hour of sleep per day, fell asleep faster, and reported higher sleep quality than their sedentary counterparts.

➤ *Avoid the use of sleeping pills.* While people over the age of 65 years comprise only 13 percent of the U.S. population, they receive 30 percent of all prescriptions for sleeping pills—which tells us that physicians are far too quick to prescribe medication when lifestyle changes and social interaction may be what's called for.

➤ *Time your naps with care.* Without question, napping on a regular basis is important in late life because of the difficulty many people have with falling and staying asleep at night. However, it's also important to limit napping, get plenty of exercise, and remain involved and engaged in life. Together, those habits should help to greatly improve nighttime sleep.

You've now made it through the entire life cycle, from infancy to old age, and read about how sleep patterns change as new challenges arise. In previous chapters, you've gained insight into some of the most common sleep problems and the best ways we know about treating them. We trust you're sleeping better already!

But there's one subject related to sleep we haven't yet focused on—and that's dreaming. We all do it: Every time we sleep for longer than about an hour, from the time we're born (maybe even from an early fetal stage) until we die, we dream. In the next chapter, we provide a brief exploration of the world of dreams and what they may—or may not—mean.

The Least You Need to Know

➤ Aging brings many changes to the body, including a disruption of sleep patterns.

➤ The aging of the biological clock may be responsible for some of the changes in sleep patterns in late life.

➤ Lifestyle factors, such as decreased physical activity, less structure, and a poor diet, often contribute to sleep problems in older people.

➤ Medical illnesses and the medications used to treat them often cause sleep problems.

➤ The best way to improve your sleep as you age is by maintaining proper sleep hygiene and healthy habits.

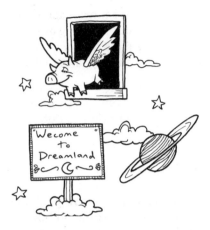

Chapter 23

The World of Dreams

In This Chapter

➤ What happens in your brain when you dream

➤ Understanding the symbolic and neurobiological meanings of dreams

➤ Learning to boost your dream recall

No book about sleep would be complete without a chapter on dreams, which are a rather fundamental part of the human experience but phenomena that remain pretty much of a mystery to even the most dedicated sleep and dream researchers.

What are dreams? Do they hold meaning to the individual who dreams them or to the culture as a whole? Why do we dream? What purpose do dreams serve to the brain, physiologically speaking? Psychologically speaking?

"Dreams are a part of nature, which harbors no intention to deceive but expresses something as best it can, just as a plant grows or an animal seeks its food..." So wrote psychoanalyst Carl Jung, a man who brought new meaning to the concept of dreams in the early part of this century. We'll discuss more about Jung's theory of dreams later, but the essence of this statement is true: Dreams *are* a part of nature. You dream, your child dreams, your cat dreams. Why we all dream, and what those dreams may mean, however, is still the subject of debate.

What about you? Do you recall your dreams and try to analyze them? Do they help you think about your life in a different way, or are they simply interesting internal "movies" that provide you with a little entertainment but nothing more?

In this chapter, we'll offer some basic information about what's known about dreams and discuss some of the many theories about their purpose and meaning as they developed in different cultures and throughout history. We'll even show you how to boost your recall of your own dreams so that you can start thinking about what they might mean to your life in a new way.

First, let's find out what we know about the physiology of dreams—what happens in the brain when you dream—to see if that could shed some light on what dreams really are.

A Quarter of the Night

As you may remember from Chapter 2, most dreaming takes place during the REM stage of sleep, which occurs about four to six times a night depending on how long you sleep. Each REM stage lasts from 10 minutes or less in the early part of the night to about 30 minutes or longer at the end of the night. Altogether, you dream for about 90 to 120 minutes, making up about 20–25 percent of your total sleep time.

Although you're asleep, your brain and body are pretty busy while you're dreaming. After spending up an hour in deep, restful sleep in which your brain waves, heart rate, and blood pressure slow down, you enter REM sleep, with each of these physiological activities speeding up and becoming irregular. In fact, on an EEG read-out of brain activity, it almost looks like you're awake. One major difference between waking and dreaming, however, is that your muscles can barely move when you're dreaming. This is apparently to keep you from acting out your dreams. That's why REM sleep is also called paradoxical sleep—your nervous system is at its highest level of activity while your body's motor system is essentially paralyzed.

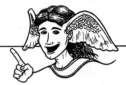

Morpheus Says

Although most dreams occur during REM sleep, you can also dream during NREM sleep stages as well. Most studies indicate that about 75 to 80 percent of people woken up from REM sleep report dreams, while only about 7 to 9 percent of people report dreams in NREM sleep. NREM dreams tend to be less vivid, active, and bizarre than REM dreams, but there appears to be some overlap in content and quality between the two, depending on the individual dreamer.

Since the discovery of REM sleep, sleep researchers have tried to locate the area of the brain responsible for REM sleep and dreaming. They believe that the brain stem, the area of the brain responsible for many basic physiological functions such as respiration, generates REM sleep. Messages to and from the brain stem and the *cerebral cortex*, the portion of the brain responsible for higher intellectual functions and certain aspects of memory, help to produce the often complex dream imagery.

Although we know something about how REM occurs in the brain, we still don't know *why* it occurs. It seems obvious that REM sleep must serve some vital function. If you're deprived of sleep one night, you make up for the loss of REM sleep the next, indicating that it's something your body needs on a regular basis, like food and water. (In laboratory studies with rats, complete deprivation of REM sleep for periods of weeks results in death, although the connection may not be a direct one.)

One theory is that REM sleep is required for learning and the processing of memory. The fact that infants spend more than 6 hours a day in REM sleep—more than three times the adult amount—supports the hypothesis that REM stimulates the brain and aids in its development. Later, as we age, the neuronal activity during REM may help maintain neuronal connections, as well as help stimulate the brain to recover from NREM sleep, in which brain activity is very low.

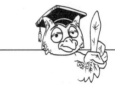

Night Owl Wisdom

The **cerebral cortex** is the intricately folded outer layer of the brain that makes up some 40 percent of its volume and is composed of an estimated 15 billion neurons. This is the part of the brain most directly responsible for consciousness.

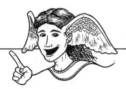

Morpheus Says

Most mammals have REM sleep and thus, the theory goes, dream. Strangely enough, opossums and ferrets hold the record for the most REM sleep, having more than 6 hours of REM sleep each day (about equal to a human newborn) and devoting more than 30 percent of their sleep time to REM sleep. Animals with very low REM sleep include elephants and hippopotami. Two mammals that never dream—or at least experience no REM sleep—are the spiny anteater of Australia and the bottle-nosed dolphin.

Well, while these theories may help start to explain the physiology of REM sleep, they certainly don't shed any light on *dreams*—those often magical, sometimes frightening, forays into what seems like another world. What exactly are dreams, and why do we have them? To find the answer to those questions, we look not only to neurobiologists—and we'll get to their theories later—but to psychologists, philosophers, artists, poets...and, well, dreamers.

The Meaning of Dreams

People have been trying to figure out the meaning and purpose of dreams since the beginning of history, and each culture has developed its own explanation for the phenomenon of dreaming. According to many traditional societies past and present, dreams can predict the future and allow contact between mortals and supernatural figures such as gods and spirits. Both the Old and the New Testament contain many significant references to dreams, as do the Islamic texts. In fact, some cultures value dreams so much that they've developed elaborate rituals to encourage dreaming, such as fasting, meditating, and choosing special places in which to sleep. In some cultures, the world of dreams takes on a reality as great as the waking world. As the *Encyclopedia of Sleep and Dreaming* (Macmillan, 1995) reports, the Chinese philosopher Chuang Tzu pointed out this connection quite succinctly when he wrote: "If I wake from a dream that I am a butterfly, am I a man who has dreamed he was a butterfly or a butterfly dreaming that I am a man?"

In modern Western culture, dream references are just as frequent. They generally focus on the psychological aspects of dreaming, with the idea that dreams offer a way to resolve personal issues and struggles. The Surrealistic school of painting, which emerged in the 1920s, represents the most direct connection between art and dreams. The Surrealists sought to fuse the dreaming and waking experiences; just take a look at the paintings of Henri Rousseau, Salvador Dali, and Joan Miro for an idea of what dreams look like to the artist, and what they symbolize to a culture.

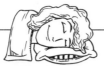

Sleep on it

Reading about the cultural aspects of dreams and dreaming is a fascinating exercise, and one that might even help you gain insight into your own dreams and what role they play in your life.

The Surrealists borrowed some of their ideas about dreams from a young Austrian psychoanalyst named Sigmund Freud, whose theories about the meaning of dreams—and about human behavior in general—were in the process of changing the world. His seminal work, *The Interpretation of Dreams*, burst onto the scene in 1900, putting a whole new spin on the new century.

The Freudian Analysis

"The interpretation of dreams is the royal road to a knowledge of the unconscious activities of the mind." So wrote Sigmund Freud, the undisputed father of modern

Western dream analysis. To Freud, dreams serve as a way to better understand ourselves, and to explore our inner urges and desires.

Freud saw the mind as being divided into the subconscious, which he called the *id*—a place of chaos and basic urges—and the conscious mind, called the *ego*, which imposes order and reason on our thoughts. He called the conscience, the judge of good and evil, the *superego*.

Freud suggested that during our waking life, the ego maintains order and morality in our minds and suppresses the desires of the id. During sleep, however, the ego relaxes its control and the id makes its desires known through dreams. Dreams thus act as a kind of safety valve for the expression of forbidden impulses. We can gratify the sexual and aggressive urges in our dreams that we cannot, due to social and moral strictures, indulge in our waking life. Freud concluded, then, that dreams are essentially wish fulfillment.

In Freud's view, another purpose of dreams is to preserve sleep. The content of dreams is often bizarre and symbolic rather than literal because the conscious mind would otherwise wake up when confronted with such disturbing experiences. In order for us to stay asleep, the unconscious expresses these wishes and fantasy in a largely disguised form—one that requires interpretation by a professional (like Freud himself) to understand. Dreams thus have both a manifest (what they seem to be) and a latent (what they really mean) content.

To help him figure out what his patients' dreams truly represented, Freud encouraged them to free associate, to simply say what first came to mind about each image or action in the dream. When the manifest dream was analyzed by the method of free association, the dream could be understood as an attempt at wish fulfillment.

The source of the content of your dreams—the body sensations, thoughts, feelings, ideas, and memories—comes from what Freud called "day residues," incomplete thoughts or tasks from the previous day that are unresolved. The latent dream thoughts, stirred by the day residues, seek some sort of expression that Freud called "dream work." There are five types of dream work, including:

Night Owl Wisdom

According to Sigmund Freud, the **id** is the instinctual, subconscious part of our psyche, while the **ego** is the conscious self that experiences and maintains contact with reality. The **superego** moderates between the instinctual drives and our sense of prohibition against them.

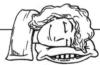

Sleep on it

The next time you remember a dream, write it down as quickly and accurately as possible. Then, for just 10 minutes, jot down any words, terms, memories, or images that spring to mind when you think of the dream. What do your thoughts tell you about the dream and why you dreamt it?

➤ *Secondary process.* This is the way we manage to make a whole story from the content of the dream, however disjointed or bizarre that content may be. You construct a story around the images of, say, your taking a bath with Sigmund or Anna Freud, your cat (who's wearing a slip) drinking out of the sink, and your mother calling you on the telephone. The thing is, according to Freud, the story you come up with actually disguises what the dream is really about.

➤ *Condensation.* Condensation refers to the tendency to combine a number of latent dream thoughts into a more succinct element. Let's say you dream of the time your high school boyfriend dumped you. Depending on other dream content, Freud might say that the boyfriend actually represents all the men in your life, including your father.

➤ *Displacement.* Displacement refers to the way we can reduce our anxieties by dreaming about them in a safe way. Maybe you're very angry with your best friend, but aren't fully aware of your feelings. You dream not of throttling your friend, but of learning that Mick Jagger (who happens to be her favorite musical artist) has lost his voice. That's displacement.

➤ *Projection.* Projection is similar to displacement, but reduces the process a step. You might dream of your best friend being killed, but you wouldn't be the one wielding the deadly weapon.

➤ *Symbolization (also known as plastic representations).* Symbolization refers to the tendency to depict a psychologically important person, body part, or experience by a repertoire of common symbols. If you dream of a knife, for instance, Freud might say you're really dreaming of a penis. A king or president in a dream might represent your father (or your psychiatrist!).

Wake Up!

You know the saying "A little knowledge can be a dangerous thing?" Well, that's especially true when it comes to interpreting your own dreams. Hunting for hidden meanings can be an interesting way to explore your feelings and hopes, but you probably should seek the advice of a professional before drawing any firm conclusions.

Clearly, interpreting your dreams according to Freudian precepts is not an easy process; in fact, Freudian analysts go through years of training before they're ready to do so. But even simply reading about the methods of interpretation can help you explore the meaning of your dreams.

Freud's theories about dreaming—and about the id and the ego in general—have fallen somewhat into disfavor in recent years, perhaps because of his insistence that all roads lead to repressed feelings of sexuality and other hidden desires. When it comes to interpreting dreams, many people look instead to one of his disciples, Carl Jung, for inspiration.

According to Jung

Once a close colleague with Freud, Swiss psychologist Carl Jung developed the branch of psychology called analytic psychology, which is heavily influenced by myth, mysticism, religion, metaphysics, and symbolism. Jung believed that dreams represented not only the repressed wishes and fantasies of the individual, but also such higher motivational drives as creativity and spirituality. According to Jung, our dreams not only reveal our true desires, anxieties, and problems, but also show us a way to resolve them.

For Jung, the *collective unconscious* was the deepest area of the mind, a sort of common psychological pool dipped into by everyone in the world. He took a profound interest in the great myths and legends of mankind and in the symbols used in the world's religions. He believed that dreams were the key to discovering and exploring the higher levels of consciousness, spirituality, and love.

Jung claimed that the collective unconscious was made up of primordial images innate in the human mind, which he called *archetypes*. We inherit these archetypes the way we inherit our eye color and intellectual capabilities. And, by understanding the archetypes, we can translate the images of our dreams and understand their language. The six primary archetypes are as follows:

Night Owl Wisdom

Archetypes are the universal psychic images that underlie all human thought. They spring from the *collective unconscious*, a concept coined by Carl Jung to define the cultural wellspring of memory.

➤ *The persona.* The image we present to the world and not our "real self," the persona appears in dreams as a person of some kind, either ourselves or someone else. If we confuse persona and real self, it can appear as an undesirable figure. Being naked in a dream can symbolize the loss of persona.

➤ *The shadow.* The shadow is the instinctive or weaker side of our nature. It provokes negative reactions such as fear and anger. Its appearance in dreams can suggest we need to exercise more control over our weaknesses.

➤ *The anima and animus.* The feminine and masculine aspects of everyone's personality are called the anima and animus. The anima is the feminine qualities in men, often represented by a beautiful or goddess-like figure. The animus is the masculine qualities in women, represented in dreams by a god-like, heroic, or powerful man.

➤ *The divine child.* Jung defined the child within, a symbol of the true self, as the divine child. The appearance of a baby or child in a dream suggests vulnerability, but also freshness, spontaneity, and potential.

➤ *The wise old man.* Symbolized by a father, priest, or other figure of authority, the appearance of the wise old man in a dream can represent the self. But he is also seen as a "mana," a powerful figure who could guide us toward the higher self as well as lead us away from it.

251

➤ *The great mother.* The great mother is a symbol not only of growth, nurturing and fertility, but also of seduction, possession, and dominance. The great mother appears in many forms: mother, princess, or witch.

As is true with Freudian dream analysis, understanding your dreams from a Jungian perspective isn't easy or straightforward. It's fun to practice, however, by trying to compare the characters and images in your dreams to these essential archetypes.

Freud and Jung are not the only psychologists who developed theories about dream and dreaming. Fritz Perls is the founder of Gestalt psychology, a type of therapy that focuses on integrating emotions and feelings into harmony in the here and now. According to Perls, dream interpretation must start from the point that all characters and objects in the dream are in fact symbols, projections of ourselves and of the way we live our lives. Dream symbolism in this view is very personal, intimately connected to our life experiences rather than either Freud's innate instinctive drives or Jung's collective unconscious.

Now that you've read about the potential symbolic meaning of dreams, it's time you learned what the neurobiologists—the scientists who study this form of brain activity from a very different perspective—have to say.

Dreams as Computer Processing

In 1964, two British scientists, Christopher Riche Evans and computer expert Edgar Arthur Newman, presented one of the earliest post-Freudian, post-Jungian dream theories. Their paper, published in *New Scientist* and titled "Dreaming: An Analogy from Computers," postulated that the brain is nothing more than an organic computer, and—just like a computer—gets cluttered with useless information. Just as a computer requires routine ridding of unwanted junk, so too does our brain need periodic tidying up.

Dreams, according to this theory, are the process by which the sleeping brain moves information worth preserving into its long-term memory, and erases from short-term memory the trivia that would otherwise clog neural pathways. As the brain cleans itself up, it activates brain cells that call up patterns and images more or less at random. Our unconscious brain does its best to put these images into some sort of coherent scenario, but because they're randomly accessed, they are usually often bizarre and nonsensical. Although they are influenced by hopes and fears, they are essentially meaningless side-effects of the cleaning-up process.

In the early 1980s, Francis Crick (who won the Nobel Prize for his role in discovering the structure of DNA) and mathematician Graeme Mitchison proposed a similar dream theory. They postulated that dreaming allows the brain to rid itself of the useless, unwanted memories that form through accidental connections between the billions of brain cells.

Finally, Allan Hobson, a psychiatry professor at Harvard Medical School added his two cents in *The Dreaming Brain* (Basic Books, 1989). According to Hobson, dreams occur as the brain uses its electrical energy to fire neurons more or less randomly while we sleep. Their meanings are transparent, in that they are naturally influenced by recent events, old memories, body states, and strong moods or desires.

What do you think? Do dreams pave the way to the unconscious? Can they help you learn about yourself, about your hopes and dreams, your problems and their solutions? Or do they represent straightforward but random firings of the brain's electrical system?

And what about the dark side of dreams? What about the things you dream about that wake you up, screaming and sweating? What kind of cleaning up could the brain be doing when that happens?

Stephen King Territory

Nightmares. Almost everyone has them at some time or another, usually during childhood. According to some statistics, nearly all children aged three to six years experience at least a few nightmares. Although they become less frequent with age, nightmares are by no means rare. The average college student experiences four to eight nightmares a year, and the average adult perhaps one or two per year. And about 5 percent of adults report having frequent nightmares—one or two per week over long periods.

Nightmares are frightening dreams that occur during REM sleep. They are almost always long, vivid dreams that contain images, actions, or outcomes that are frightening or anxiety-provoking in the dreamer. Usually, nightmares involve being chased or threatened by either a person or, mostly in the case of children, a monster or wild animal.

Why do nightmares occur? It may be better to ask *when* they occur, which is almost always during times of stress and change. The loss of a loved one to death or divorce, a change in career, an accident or other trauma—any and all of these events can trigger a nightmare.

Like all other dreams, nightmares come from the mind of the dreamer, and therefore reflect in some way the dreamer's memories, problems, wishes, and fears. And, just like other dreams, they can be interpreted using the theories of Freud, Jung, Perls, or others.

Wake Up!

Nightmares are almost always benign occurrences that do not require either medical or psychological treatment. However, if you're having recurring nightmares that frequently disturb your sleep, you may want to talk to your doctor or a therapist about them. Your fears and anxieties may be getting the best of you, and you may need some help in resolving them.

Boosting Your Dream Power

Before you can attempt to figure out what your dreams may or may not mean, you need to remember them as clearly and accurately as possible. Unfortunately, dreams are among the more fleeting experiences known to man or woman: Within seconds of waking up from a dream, most of us start to forget all but the most dramatic or meaningful images.

Here are a few tips to help you remember your dreams:

➤ *Get plenty of sleep.* The more rested you are, the easier it will be to focus on your goal of recalling dreams. In addition, dream periods get longer and closer together as the night progresses—the more you sleep, the more likely you are to experience a long dream worth remembering!

➤ *Maintain a dream journal.* Keep a notebook and pen next to your bed and record every dream you remember, no matter how disjointed or strange. Even if all you remember is a face or a room or a feeling, write it down. And record it right away, even if you wake up in the middle of the night. Otherwise, you're apt to forget it by morning.

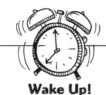

Wake Up!

If you believe the "computer clean-up" theory of dreaming, you may not *want* to remember your dreams. That is, if you think the brain dreams in order to rid itself of extraneous bits of useless information that otherwise would clog it up and slow it down, you might be best served by letting them pass from your memory altogether.

➤ *Remind yourself that you want to remember your dreams as you fall asleep.* Some people report that they're better able to recall their dreams if they concentrate on doing so as they fall asleep. It's especially helpful, according to this method, if you do so while practicing one of the relaxation methods we mentioned in Chapter 8. If you're performing progressive relaxation, for instance, you can think "I will dream and remember my dreams" each time you relax a muscle group. You may find yourself better able to recall your dreams when you wake up.

➤ *Time your wake-up call.* As you may remember, you dream about every 90 minutes at the end of each sleep cycle. Try setting your alarm clock for $7^1/_2$ hours (five full cycles) past the time you normally fall asleep. That way, you might be lucky enough to wake up after your longest and most fully realized dream of the night.

Well there you have it. Now you know not only all about sleep and how to improve your chances of sleeping well, but a little bit about one of the mysterious "side effects" of sleep: your dreams.

We hope you're already starting to improve your sleep habits and, by doing so, getting a better night's sleep. In the next section, we offer you some further resources should you want or need more information about sleep. In the meantime, we wish you all a good night.

The Least You Need to Know

➤ Your brain is working very hard as it produces the dreams you dream at night.

➤ Sigmund Freud thought the content of our dreams reflected unconscious and repressed desires and needs.

➤ Carl Jung interpreted dreams using archetypes—universal symbols taken from our individual self and from our collective unconscious.

➤ Dreams may be nothing more than random, electrical signals in the brain.

➤ You can boost your recall of dreams by concentrating on remembering them before you go to sleep.

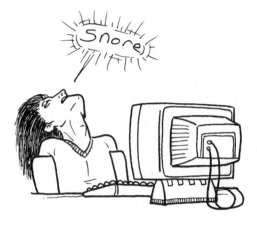

More Sleep Promoters

More, more, more: That's probably what you're asking for right now, isn't it? Well, we certainly hope we've whet your appetite for information about the world of sleep, or at least identified some of the specific challenges you face when it comes to sleeping well.

In this section, we offer you a list of associations involved in sleep and sleep research, as well as a list of books on the subject that might interest you.

Associations and Organizations

The associations offer information, most of it free, about different aspects of sleep and sleep disorders. In addition to their addresses and phone numbers, we also provide (where possible) their Internet addresses. Please be advised, however, that many Web pages offer links to other sources of information, and that not all of these sources are reputable. Circadian Technologies (listed below) has a nifty page of Web links from its own Web site that is always kept up-to-date, so you may want to start there.

In addition, make sure you talk to your doctor or other appropriately informed and licensed health care professional about any issue, treatment, or theory that interests you before making changes in your health habits.

Circadian Technologies, Inc.
125 Cambridge Park Dr.
Cambridge, MA 02140
(617) 492-5060
Internet address: http://www.circadian.com

CTI helps individuals and companies cope with the sleep and alertness problems that arise when people work outside the traditional hours of 9 to 5, or sleep during the day instead of the night. The research, consulting services and publications of CTI help companies and their employees cope effectively with living and working in our modern 24-hour society. These services introduce optimal practices and technologies to prevent sleep disruption and fatigue, human error and accidents, poor mood and morale, reduced productivity and creativity, and impaired health in multi-shift or global operations.

Dr. Martin Moore-Ede formed the company in 1983 as an outgrowth of his research on sleep, alertness and biological clocks at Harvard Medical School. CTI works with all levels of organizations from its offices in Boston, London, and elsewhere, and provides:

➤ *Global Travel Policies*: Programs in fatigue, stress and jet lag management for the executives and senior managers of global corporations with significant travel commitments

➤ *Fatigue Management Programs*: Installation of comprehensive corporate Alertness Assurance programs in the around-the-clock operations of *transportation* (aviation, railroad, transit, marine, trucking), *industrial* (manufacturing, chemical, oil, utility, paper, mining, semiconductor, etc.), and *service* operations (health care, financial, telecommunication, security and military) to eliminate the risks of fatigue

➤ *Sleep Disorder Screening and Treatment*: Confidential screening programs to identify and treat employees with sleep apnea and other sleep disorders

➤ *Shift Scheduling*: Development and installation of shift schedules and work assignments that optimize employee alertness, performance and health, while meeting their personal needs for quality sleep and off-duty time

➤ *Training*: Tailored programs in sleep and alertness management, to address the needs of individuals and organizations using Individual, Group, Train-the-trainer, CD-ROM, videotape, Internet and other media

➤ *Publications*: Circadian Information, an affiliate of CTI, publishes and distributes books, training materials, videotapes, newsletters including *Working Nights*, *Shiftwork Alert*, and *Briefing on Shiftwork*, and the free Web site Circadian Learning Center at www.circadian.com

➤ *Research and Technology Development*: The Circadian Alertness Laboratory, a division of CTI, conducts assessments of fatigue risk, benchmarking of multi-shift operations, development of new fatigue countermeasures, evaluations of equipment effectiveness in alertness measurement, and measurement of program outcome

The American Sleep Disorders Association

6301 Bandel Rd., Suite 101
Rochester, MN 55901
(507) 287-6006
Internet address: http://www.asda.org/

Known as the ASDA, this professional medical organization has a membership made up of nearly 300 sleep disorders centers across the country and more than 3,400 clinicians and researchers. It establishes standards for evaluating and treating sleep disorders, as well as promoting education, training, and research in sleep disorders medicine. It represents the sleep disorders discipline before health regulatory agencies and other health organizations. The ASDA Web site includes information directed toward both clinicians and the general public, and offers access to a series of wellness booklets about sleep and sleep disorders.

The National Sleep Foundation
729 Fifteenth St. NW, 4th Floor
Washington, DC 20005
Internet address: http://www.sleepfoundation.org

The National Sleep Foundation is a nonprofit organization that promotes public understanding of sleep and sleep disorders and supports sleep-related education, research, and advocacy to improve public health and safety. It publishes two magazines, the bimonthly *Sleep Medicine Alert* and the quarterly *The NSF Connection,* as well as a variety of reports and brochures. Its Web site is full of invaluable information for interested sleepers (or wanna be sleepers!), including up-to-date information on sleep, sleep deprivation, and sleep disorders and their treatment.

The American Sleep Apnea Association
2025 Pennsylvania Ave. NW, Suite 905
Washington, DC 20006
Internet address: http://www.sleepapnea.org

A nonprofit organization, the American Sleep Apnea Association (ASAA) is dedicated to reducing injury, disability, and death from sleep apnea and to enhancing the well-being of those affected by this common disorder. It offers booklets and pamphlets to interested consumers, as well as the A.W.A.K.E. network of support groups for affected patients in 45 states.

The Narcolepsy Network
P.O. Box 1365
FDR Station
New York, NY 10150
Internet address: http://www.Websciences.org/narnet/

The Narcolepsy Network is a national, nonprofit organization for people who have narcolepsy (or related sleep disorders), their families and friends, and professionals involved in treatment, research, and public education about narcolepsy. It offers educational publications, audio and videotapes, and other material to those interested.

Light Sources

In Chapter 11 (and elsewhere), we discussed the uses of artificial light sources in the treatment of sleep disorders and other conditions, including jet lag, problems related to shift work, and Seasonal Affective Disorder. Here, we list some of the reputable manufacturers and retailers of artificial light sources.

Environmental Lighting Concepts, Inc.
3923 Coconut Palm Dr., #101
Tampa, FL 33619
(800) 842-8848

OTT BioLightSystems, Inc.
28 Parker Way
Santa Barbara, CA 93101
(800) 234-3724
Internet address: ott@silcom.com

Duro-test
9 Law Dr.
Fairfield, NJ 07004
(973) 808-6622

The SunBox Company
19217 Orbit Dr.
(800) LITE-YOU
Internet address: sunbox@aol.com

Bio-Brite, Inc.
7315 Wisconsin Ave. #1300W
Bethesda, MD 20814
(800) 621-LITE
Internet address: biobrite@aol.com

Enviro-Med
1600 SE 141st Ave.
Vancouver, WA 98684
(800) 222-DAWN

Further Reading

Alvarez, A. *Night: Night Life, Night Language, Sleep, and Dreams*. New York: W.W. Norton, 1995.

Anthony, William, A. *The Art of Napping*. New York: Larson Publications, 1997.

Buchman, Dian Dincin. *The Complete Guide to Natural Sleep*. New Canaan, CT: Keats, 1997.

Carskadon, Mary A. (ed.). *The Encyclopedia of Sleep and Dreaming*. New York: Macmillan, 1995.

Coren, Stanley. *Sleep Thieves*. New York: The Free Press, 1996.

Dement, William C. *The Sleepwatchers*. Palo Alto, CA: Stanford Alumni Association, 1992.

Ferber, Richard. *Solve Your Child's Sleep Problems*. New York: Simon and Schuster, 1985.

Fontana, David. *The Secret Power of Dreams*. Rockport, MA: Element, 1990.

Freud, Sigmund. *The Interpretation of Dreams*. New York: Penguin, 1976.

Gottlieb, Susan E. *Keys to Children's Sleep Problems*. New York: Barron's, 1993.

Hauri, Peter. *No More Sleepless Nights*. New York: John Wiley & Sons, 1990.

Hobson, Allan J. *The Dreaming Brain*. New York: Basic Books, 1988.

Hobson, Allan J. *Sleep*. New York: Basic Books, 1989.

Lavie, Peretz. *The Enchanted World of Sleep*. New Haven, CT: Yale University Press, 1996.

Maas, James B. *Power Sleep*. New York: Villard, 1998.

Moore-Ede, Martin. *The 24-Hour Society*. New York: Addison-Wesley, 1993.

Zammit, Gary. *Good Nights*. Kansas City: Andrews and McMeel, 1997.

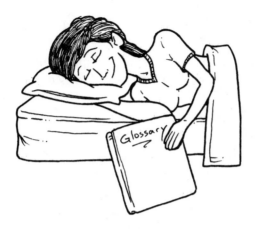

Glossary

Unless you've delved into the world of sleep in the past, reading this book probably opened your eyes to a variety of new concepts about sleep and body rhythms, ones that had some words and terms that may have been unfamiliar to you. We hope the following glossary of terms helps you on your journey to a good night's sleep.

Alzheimer's disease: A type of dementia; a progressive degeneration of the brain that occurs in about 5 to 10 percent of the population over the age of 65. Like many other brain disorders, Alzheimer's disease may cause sleep disturbances.

Apnea: From the Greek word *pnoia* meaning "breath" and the Greek prefix *a* denoting "absence"; apnea is the temporary cessation of breathing for any reason. *Obstructive Sleep Apnea* is a common sleep disorder.

Automatic behavior: A phenomenon reported by the sleep deprived in which they perform relatively routine behavior without having any memory of doing so. Automatic behavior can be quite dangerous if the behavior involves driving an automobile or performing a routine but sensitive task at work.

Autonomic nervous system: The part of the nervous system responsible for largely unconscious bodily functions such as the heartbeat, blood pressure, and digestion. It is divided into two divisions, the sympathetic and parasympathetic.

Biofeedback: A behavior modification therapy in which patients are taught to control bodily functions such as blood pressure and heart rate through conscious effort. Biofeedback can be especially helpful in learning to reduce stress.

Brain stem: The part of the nervous system located at the base of the brain, connecting the spinal cord with the rest of the brain; containing essential mechanisms that regulate sleep/wake behavior.

Cataplexy: Sudden spell of weakness—often related to an intense emotional reaction—due to a decrease in muscle tone. Cataplexy is one of the most important symptoms of *narcolepsy*.

Chronobiology: The study of the biological clocks used by humans and other living things to keep time, and the biological rhythms these clocks maintain.

Chronotherapy: A specific treatment method devised to correct disruptions of circadian rhythms, particularly the sleep disorders *Delayed Sleep Phase Syndrome*, *Advanced Sleep Phase Syndrome*, and related problems.

Circadian rhythm: From the Latin *circa*, meaning "about" and *dies*, meaning "day," a circadian rhythm is a biological event that regularly recurs about every 24 hours.

Colic: A problem that occurs in infants involving long crying spells. Colic may disrupt the sleep patterns of both parent and child.

Continuous Positive Airway Pressure (CPAP): Treatment for *Obstructive Sleep Apnea* that works by reversing the negative pressure that causes the throat to collapse during sleep. A machine pumps air through a plastic mask that fits over the nose. The air pressure holds the throat open, which allows for continuous breathing and prevents the frequent awakening suffered by most people with Obstructive Sleep Apnea.

Cortisol: A steroid hormone produced by the adrenal glands that affects metabolism, the stress response, and the process of inflammation. Like other hormones, cortisol is released in the body with a circadian rhythm.

Delayed Sleep Phase Disorder (DSPS): Sleep disorder characterized by the inability to fall asleep and awaken according to ordinary schedules. Typically, the affected person is unable to fall asleep until 3 or 4 a.m. and finds it difficult to awaken earlier than 10 or 11 a.m. Once asleep, however, someone with DSPS sleeps normally.

Dementia: A term used to describe any number of conditions that involve a generalized, progressive, and usually irreversible deterioration of memory and cognition. One type of age-related dementia is *Alzheimer's disease*. Most, if not all, types of dementia cause sleep problems.

Depression: A mental disorder that often involves feelings of sadness and despair, but also slowed thinking, decreased pleasure, appetite changes, physical aches and pains, and sleeping difficulties.

Electroencephalograph (EEG): A recording of the electrical signals generated by the brain; frequently used by sleep researchers to evaluate sleep patterns and identify potential sleep disorders.

Electromyogram (EMG): A recording of the electrical signals created when muscle fibers contract. Used by sleep researchers to detect the movements associated with certain sleep stages and sleep disorders.

Electrooculograph (EOG): A recording of eye movements during sleep.

Endogenous: A word used to describe a rhythm or condition that arises within the body and is not caused or triggered by external or environmental factors.

Entrainment: Term used by sleep researchers to describe the process by which internal biological rhythms such as sleep/wake patterns become synchronized to external *Zeitgebers*.

Free running: Term used in *chronobiology* indicating a biological rhythm running on its own spontaneous rhythm no longer synchronized with the environment.

Human growth hormone: Body chemical secreted by the pituitary gland during deep, non-REM sleep that works to promote body growth and repair.

Hypnagogic hallucination: A dream-like experience that occurs in the interval between wakefulness and sleep; common among normal sleepers, but also one of the four classic signs of *narcolepsy*.

Hypnic jerk: Sudden spontaneous jerk of part or all of the body that occurs during the drowsy period or during light sleep, making it difficult to fall and stay asleep.

Infradian rhythm: A biological rhythm that regularly recurs with a periodicity of longer than 24 hours.

Insomnia: The inability to fall or stay asleep at the right time, for the right length of time, and with sufficient quality to feel well and alert during the day.

Internal desynchronization: The loss of synchrony among two or more internal *circadian rhythms*; a frequent side effect of jet lag.

Jet lag: Maladjustment experienced when travel across time zones results in an abrupt change in the length of day. This causes body time to become out of synch with local clock time.

Lark: A person whose natural rhythms causes him or her to prefer the early morning hours for activity and concentration, and who prefers to go to bed fairly early in the evenings.

Light therapy: A procedure for treating *Seasonal Affective Disorder* and other disorders related to length of day, exposure to daylight, or shifts in circadian rhythms, including Delayed Phase Sleep Disorder (DSPS), Advanced Phase Disorder (ASPS), jet lag and some shift work. Involves exposure to bright light at specific times in order to shift the biological clock or to maintain rhythms that may otherwise be lost.

Melatonin: A hormone released into the bloodstream by the *pineal gland*, which is stimulated by darkness and prohibited by light.

Microsleep: A very brief (less than 30-second), involuntary episode of sleep that occurs during ongoing wakeful activity. A frequent symptom of extreme sleep deprivation.

Multiple Sleep Latency Test: A test used to measure how long it takes for a person to fall asleep during the day, and thus a person's daytime level of sleepiness and sleep deprivation.

Narcolepsy: A sleep disorder characterized by excessive, irresistible daytime sleepiness that causes someone to fall asleep at inappropriate times. Other symptoms include *cataplexy, sleep paralysis,* and *hypnagogic hallucinations.*

Nightmare: A frightening dream that one remembers or the experience of awakening feeling frightened. Nightmares occur during *REM sleep.*

Night terror: A phenomenon occurring in deep sleep in which the person is terrified and often screaming and sitting up in bed and even sleepwalking.

Night owl: Someone whose natural rhythms cause them to prefer staying up late at night and avoiding the morning hours. A night owl generally feels most alert and competent in the evening.

NREM sleep: Non-Rapid Eye Movement sleep include Stages 1–4 of the sleep cycle—all but the dreaming portion of sleep.

Obstructive Sleep Apnea: A sleep disorder involving an obstruction of the air passages, particularly the airway between the nasal openings and the voice box. Symptoms include heavy snoring, frequent awakenings, and daytime sleepiness.

Parasomnia: A disturbance during sleep such as sleepwalking, sleeptalking, bedwetting, and night terrors.

Phase response curve: A graph describing the resetting of the timing of a circadian rhythm by a *Zeitgeber,* and how the shift varies in direction and length according to the time of day that the Zeitgeber is presented.

Polysomnogram: The sleep recording that displays brain activity, eye movement, and motor activity. Used by sleep researchers as a diagnostic and clinical tool.

REM sleep: Sleep characterized by rapid eye movement, brain activity close to that of wakefulness, and a complete absence of muscle tone. Most dreaming takes place during REM sleep.

REM Sleep Behavior Disorder (RBD): A disorder marked by the loss of the normal paralysis that accompanies REM sleep, marked by complex and often violent behavior that occurs while the sleeper is in REM sleep.

Seasonal Affective Disorder (SAD): A form of clinical *depression* in which a person becomes depressed every year during certain months—particularly during the fall and winter when day lengths are shorter.

Sleep cycle: The approximately 90–100 minute cyclic fluctuations containing both *REM* and *NREM* sleep.

Sleep deprivation: Term used to describe the state you're in when you don't obtain enough sleep to satisfy the needs of your body and mind. Symptoms—the severity of which depend on both how sleep deprived you are and how sensitive your body is to the loss of sleep—may include daytime sleepiness, fatigue, irritability and mood swings, itchy eyes, fatigue, appetite changes, inability to concentrate, and others.

Sleep hygiene: Those practices of daily living that promote good sleep, including eating a proper diet, getting regular exercise, creating a conducive sleep environment, and others.

Sleep inertia: The symptoms of confusion and grogginess that may occur upon awakening, especially from deep Stages 3 and 4 of sleep.

Sleep paralysis: A brief episode of partial or total paralysis occurring at the beginning or end of a sleep period, usually occurring to people with *narcolepsy*.

Sleepwalking: A *parasomnia* that involves a sleeping person who leaves the bed and walks around in or outside of the house. Also called somnambulism.

Snoring: The hoarse sound of breathing during sleep that occurs when the soft palate vibrates. Excessive snoring may indicate Obstructive Sleep Apnea, a serious and common sleep disorder.

Sudden Infant Death Syndrome: The sudden death of an infant, during sleep, with no known cause; the leading cause of death in infants between the first month and first year of life.

Sundown syndrome: The recurrent appearance of behavioral disturbances such as agitation, aggression, pacing and restlessness during the late afternoon or evening among elderly or demented patients.

Suprachiasmatic nucleus of the hypothalamus (SCN): A tiny cluster of brain cells that serve as the body's primary circadian biological clock, helping to orchestrate the sleep/wake cycle and a host of other physiological functions.

Teeth grinding: The grinding of teeth during sleep caused by tension, or a malalignment of the teeth within the jaw. Also called bruxism.

Tryptophan: One of the essential amino acids found in a variety of foods that is the precursor to *serotonin*, a known sleep promoter.

Ultradian rhythms: Biological rhythms that recur during a period shorter than 24 hours, such as the REM/NREM cycle of sleep that recurs every 90 to 100 minutes during the night.

Uvulopalatopharyngoplasty (UPPP): Surgery used to correct *Obstructive Sleep Apnea* that involves the trimming of excess tissue of the soft palate and other tissue to reconstruct the air space, allowing clear breathing during the sleep.

Zeitgeber: From the German meaning "time giver," an environmental cue (particularly light) that helps *entrain* the body's rhythm to the 24-hour day.

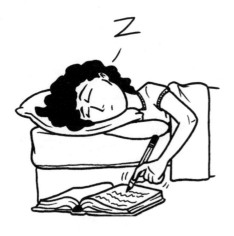

Your Sleep Log

In Chapter 5, we discussed the importance of keeping track of both the quality of your sleep and your sleep/wake patterns. To help you meet that goal, we provide here several days worth of a Sleep Log that you should fill in every day. If you like, you can use the information to fill in the Sleep Graph, found in both Chapter 5 and on the tear-out card at the front of the book. We suggest you photocopy this log and save several pages of blank Sleep Log forms so that you can continue the process in the months and years to come.

Your Sleep Log

Date _____

Worktime _____

Playtime _____

Bedtime _____

Lights Out _____

Sleep Onset _____

Awakenings:

Number/Length _____

Wake-Up Time _____

Rise Time _____

Sleep Quality (1 = terrible, 2 = poor, 3 = fair, 4 = good, 5 = very good, 6 = excellent)
_____

Nap Time/Duration _____

Date _____

Worktime _____

Playtime _____

Bedtime _____

Lights Out _____

Sleep Onset _____

Awakenings:

Number/Length _____

Wake-Up Time _____

Rise Time _____

Sleep Quality (1 = terrible, 2 = poor, 3 = fair, 4 = good, 5 = very good, 6 = excellent)
_____

Nap Time/Duration _____

Date _____

Worktime _____

Playtime _____

Bedtime _____

Lights Out _____

Sleep Onset _____

Awakenings:

Number/Length _____

Wake-Up Time _____

Rise Time _____

Sleep Quality (1 = terrible, 2 = poor, 3 = fair, 4 = good, 5 = very good, 6 = excellent)
_____

Nap Time/Duration _____

Date _____

Worktime _____

Playtime _____

Bedtime _____

Lights Out _____

Sleep Onset _____

Awakenings:

Number/Length _____

Wake-Up Time _____

Rise Time _____

Sleep Quality (1 = terrible, 2 = poor, 3 = fair, 4 = good, 5 = very good, 6 = excellent)

_____

Nap Time/Duration _____

Date _____

Worktime _____

Playtime _____

Bedtime _____

Lights Out _____

Sleep Onset _____

Awakenings:

Number/Length _____

Wake-Up Time _____

Rise Time _____

Sleep Quality (1 = terrible, 2 = poor, 3 = fair, 4 = good, 5 = very good, 6 = excellent)

_____

Nap Time/Duration _____

Date _____

Worktime _____

Playtime _____

Bedtime _____

Lights Out _____

Sleep Onset _____

Awakenings:

Number/Length _____

Wake-Up Time _____

Rise Time _____

Sleep Quality (1 = terrible, 2 = poor, 3 = fair, 4 = good, 5 = very good, 6 = excellent)
_____

Nap Time/Duration _____

Date _____

Worktime _____

Playtime _____

Bedtime _____

Lights Out _____

Sleep Onset _____

Awakenings:

Number/Length _____

Wake-Up Time _____

Rise Time _____

Sleep Quality (1 = terrible, 2 = poor, 3 = fair, 4 = good, 5 = very good, 6 = excellent)
_____

Nap Time/Duration _____

Date _____

Worktime _____

Playtime _____

Bedtime _____

Lights Out _____

Sleep Onset _____

Awakenings:

Number/Length _____

Wake-Up Time _____

Rise Time _____

Sleep Quality (1 = terrible, 2 = poor, 3 = fair, 4 = good, 5 = very good, 6 = excellent)
_____

Nap Time/Duration _____

Date _____

Worktime _____

Playtime _____

Bedtime _____

Lights Out _____

Sleep Onset _____

Awakenings:

Number/Length _____

Wake-Up Time _____

Rise Time _____

Sleep Quality (1 = terrible, 2 = poor, 3 = fair, 4 = good, 5 = very good, 6 = excellent)
_____

Nap Time/Duration _____

Date _____

Worktime _____

Playtime _____

Bedtime _____

Lights Out _____

Sleep Onset _____

Awakenings:

Number/Length _____

Wake-Up Time _____

Rise Time _____

Sleep Quality (1 = terrible, 2 = poor, 3 = fair, 4 = good, 5 = very good, 6 = excellent)
_____

Nap Time/Duration _____

Date _____

Worktime _____

Playtime _____

Bedtime _____

Lights Out _____

Sleep Onset _____

Awakenings:

Number/Length _____

Wake-Up Time _____

Rise Time _____

Sleep Quality (1 = terrible, 2 = poor, 3 = fair, 4 = good, 5 = very good, 6 = excellent)
_____

Nap Time/Duration _____

Index